greenmama

greenmama

Giving Your Child a Healthy Start and a Greener Future

Manda Aufochs Gillespie

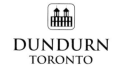

DUNDURN
TORONTO

Editor: Allison Hirst
Design: Courtney Horner
Printer: Transcontinental

Library and Archives Canada Cataloguing in Publication

Aufochs Gillespie, Manda, author
Green mama : giving your
child a healthy start and a greener future / Manda Aufochs
Gillespie.

Includes bibliographical references.
Issued in print and electronic formats.
ISBN 978-1-4597-2295-8

1. Child rearing--Environmental aspects. 2. Sustainable living.
3. Environmental health. I. Title.

HQ769.A93 2014   649'.1   C2014-901019-2
                                        C2014-901020-6

     1   2   3   4   5   18   17   16   15   14

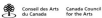 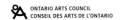

We acknowledge the support of the **Canada Council for the Arts** and the **Ontario Arts Council** for our publishing program. We also acknowledge the financial support of the **Government of Canada** through the **Canada Book Fund** and **Livres Canada Books**, and the **Government of Ontario** through the **Ontario Book Publishing Tax Credit** and the **Ontario Media Development Corporation**.

All photographs, unless otherwise indicated, are by Vanessa Zises Filley.

Cover design by Laura Boyle.

Printed and bound in Canada.

Visit us at
Dundurn.com
@dundurnpress
Facebook.com/dundurnpress
Pinterest.com/dundurnpress

Dundurn
3 Church Street, Suite 500
Toronto, Ontario, Canada
M5E 1M2

Gazelle Book Services Limited
White Cross Mills
High Town, Lancaster, England
LA1 4XS

Dundurn
2250 Military Road
Tonawanda, NY
U.S.A. 14150

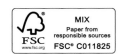

This book is dedicated to all the world's children,
especially my own beloved Zella Rose and Zada "Maela."
May we create a world worthy of them all.

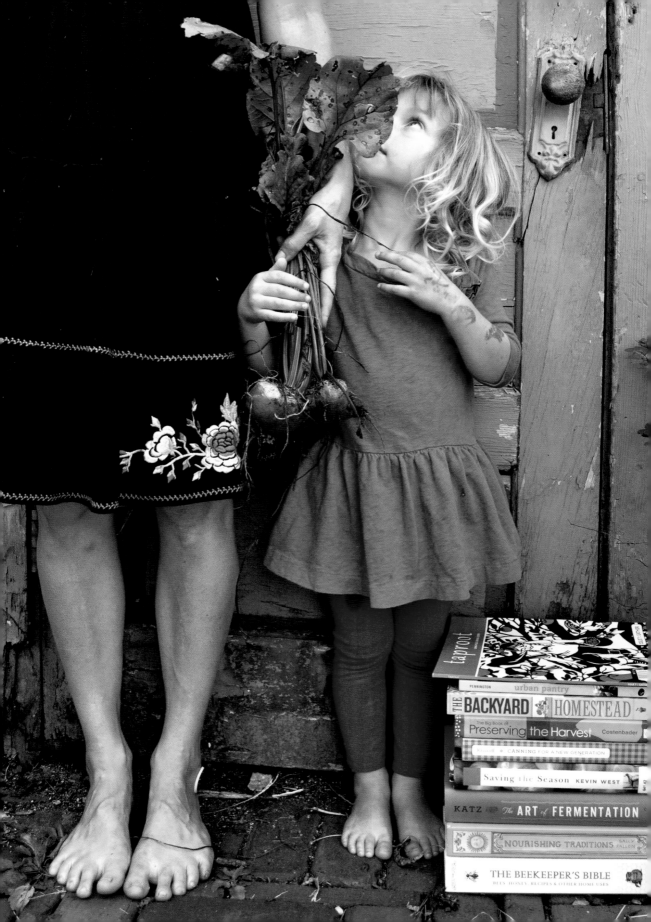

Contents

· ·

Acknowledgements

· ·

A book like this is a community effort. It draws upon the tireless work of scientists, researchers, writers, activists, and parents. In addition to those I mention in the book, I would also like to acknowledge the help of Sarah Newstok, Roxanne Engstrom, Cecelia Ungari, Nora Gainer, Bridget Felix, Maureen Gainer Reilly, Glenys Webster, and Betty Krawczyk. I would also like to thank the many parents who have allowed me a glimpse into their lives through my Green Mama work and the Green Mama helpers past, present, and (I hope) future. It is hard to express just how much you have all inspired me. Despite what might seem like depressing work at times, I am more hopeful than I have ever been. Thank you for your support, time, and love.

A few friends stand out particularly for their efforts to support this book project. Deena Chochinov sat me down and explained just how I was going to negotiate getting the time to write this book amongst the craziness of family life, other jobs, and while my husband was simultaneously writing a book. Linda Solomon Wood insisted I send my manuscript to an agent and Tzeporah Berman introduced me to the amazing agents who took it. Jill Riddell, Lynn Powell, and Jennifer Block provided early guidance. Carrie Saxifrage read every chapter, sometimes multiple times, even while she was working on her own book. Some days, after reading chapters and chapters, she would then take my eldest for a hike in the woods or force me onto my bicycle and off to *Boing!*

The photographs in the book are the generous gift of a talented artist, Vanessa Zises Filley. Not only did she coax her children, my children, and many other people's children into posing, she took this project into her heart to create photos that tell a story of love. To follow Vanessa's work, visit her at *vanessafilley.com*.

My agents, Westwood Creative Artists, have been amazing to work with. I owe gratitude in particular to Chris Casuccio for his unrelenting belief in this book and his willingness to be both friend and guide on the journey and to Hilary McMahon for sharing her extensive contacts and knowledge of publishing. I am also thankful for the entire team at Dundurn, with the faithful and talented Diane Young at the lead, the editorial support of Allison Hirst, and the numerous other creative talents who worked hard to make this book especially beautiful, accessible, and available. Thank you for believing, as I do, that parents do still read books.

This book also belongs to my family, who, knowingly or not, got me into the green mama line of work: my grandmothers, Rose Marie and Ethel Mae, the latter of whom shared some of her parenting stories and knowledge for this book; my grandfather, who would walk with me in the woods until my own love for nature was found; my mother, who planted our childhood garden in the burnt-out remains of the house next door; my father, who taught me the power of a smile; my beloved siblings, all of whom provide me with a much needed reality check while never belittling my green-craziness. And most especially I want to thank my husband, Sadhu Aufochs Johnston — that I ended up with someone as loving, inspiring, and eco-conscious as he is suggests that we do, sometimes, get more than we deserve — and my children, who have taught me to love at new depths, laugh more, and hope.

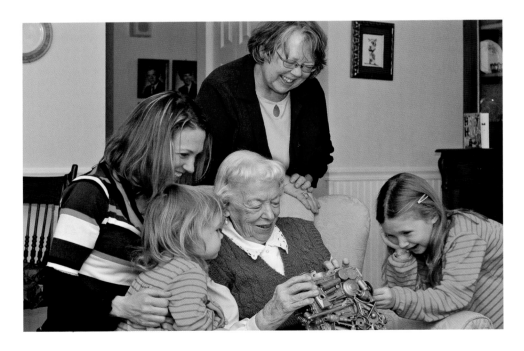

The Meaning of Green

· ·

By way of introduction, let me tell you that "green" wasn't the first thing on my mother's mind when she was raising me. She was single with three kids, no money, and little support. Her worries were immediate: How would she feed us three meals a day? Who would care for the baby while she went to school to finish her degree? How could she save enough money to move her family to a safer neighbourhood? But her parenting *was* green: She planted a garden in the burnt-out lot next door and grew fresh vegetables. Our clothes were handed down. And we never wasted anything.

Similarly, my grandmother had no concept of green — other than as a colour — but she made her family's food from scratch, cleaned the house with baking soda, vinegar, and a bit of lemon, and breastfed her babies. She rarely flew on airplanes or ate out. She prided herself on reusing, recycling, and simply using less.

The point is that what we call "green" today used to be the norm. Both my grandmother's and my mother's parenting choices were simplified by the absence of things that our generation is expected to accept as a matter of course: industrial chemicals in consumer products; computer and TV screens to pacify children; marketing aimed at kids. Back in the day, screens still hung on doors, no one had heard of climate destabilization, and, some researchers believe, the parent-child attachment was stronger, so kids were easier to parent.

Things have changed a lot, and they keep changing — fast. Many parents long for the simplicity of the time before the daunting rise in cases of ADHD, autism, asthma, diabetes, food allergies, childhood cancers, and attachment disorders; a time before North America imported or produced billions of pounds of chemicals daily. Regardless of our demographics, the increased difficulty of keeping our kids safe binds parents together.

The Crib Sheet

Confused by an acronym in the book? Here they are spelled out.

AAP	American Academy of Pediatrics
ADHD	attention deficit hyperactivity disorder
AMA	American Medical Association
BFHI	Baby-Friendly Hospital Initiative
BPA	bisphenol-A
BPS	bisphenol-S
CDC	(U.S.) Centers for Disease Control and Prevention
CMA	Canadian Medical Association
CPS	Canadian Paediatric Society
CSC	Campaign for Safer Cosmetics
EC	elimination communication
EMF	electromagnetic field
EPA	Environmental Protection Agency
EWG	Environmental Working Group
FDA	(U.S.) Food and Drug Administration
GMO (GM, GE)	genetically modified (or engineered) organism
IARC	International Agency for Research on Cancer
LLLI	La Leche League International
NRDC	National Resource Defense Council
NTP	National Toxicology Program
PBDEs	polybrominated diphenyl ethers (a flame retardant)
PVC	polyvinyl chloride (vinyl)
SAP	superabsorbent polymer
SIDS	sudden infant death syndrome
VOC	volatile organic compounds
WHO	World Health Organization

Yet there is nothing more hopeful than choosing to have a child. When we make that decision, we say "I believe the future is worth bringing a person into." We create the neurological capacity for hope. Parents by their nature get something right that many environmentalists get wrong: hope is the best motivator for change. In my work as The Green Mama, I see a combination of love and joy and longing that is born in the hearts of parents with the birth of their child. It's helped along by a stew of delicious hormones and more new neural pathways than are created at almost any other time of life. It helps explain why so many new parents get serious about going green. We always have the capacity for change, but having a baby changes everything. We will do absolutely anything to keep that baby safe.

My grandmother and mother were green because of circumstance, but when I had my kids, being green was a conscious choice that took work. I had spent my whole career greening things: more livable neighbourhoods, a multi-million-dollar residential project, and one of the few urban eco-village projects in the United States. As a researcher and writer, I also knew all sorts of facts about how far people will walk to take transit, ways cities can adapt for climate change, and the benefits of urban recycling programs.

But everything I knew about greening the larger world didn't translate into how to give my child the healthiest start in life. At first, it seemed liked everything I had ever done (according to my extensive late-night Internet browsing) was "wrong." I ate too much fish full of mercury. I exposed myself to lead when renovating my old house, slept on a toxic mattress during my pregnancy, and celebrated my conception with a visit to the nail salon. I didn't detoxify my breast milk and I used "the best" bottles, which it turned out still leached BPA. The information alarmed me, it was often contradictory, and it rarely included practical solutions for how to make things better.

I wanted a guide. But who could I ask? My fantastic and progressive doctors and midwives didn't have the time or information to answer detailed questions. There was little reliable advice on the Web and even less in parenting magazines or books. My mother and grandmother shared many of my values, yet they had parented in a much simpler world.

So I did what I had always done. I read studies, talked with scientists and mothers, and experimented. I asked: *What is the connection between the health of the world and my growing child?*

I wasn't the only one asking this question: co-workers, friends, and members of the media were increasingly "eco-curious." Soon, I was sharing my research and stories with other parents and professionals in parent groups like The Green Mama Cafe, in workshops, and in writing. When I shared my discoveries with others, I found I could relax, laugh, and find inspiration in coming together to navigate through this newly acquired knowledge.

Compared to becoming a parent, going green is easy. Indeed, going green is probably easier for new parents than for just about anybody else because our brains get rewired to form new habits. As we develop the capacity to deal with our baby's soiled diapers in the middle of the night, we can use that same malleability to learn a few other new habits as well — like sorting the recycling, doing full loads of laundry, and reading the fine print on labels. Research into the neurological and biological basis of empathy suggests that our ability to care for our children makes it easier to care about more abstract things, like the state of the world. The more we believe in that green future, the more good feelings we generate. We take hopeful actions and that generates more good feelings.

Over the years, I have met dozens of new parents who would "never" use cloth diapers, but found themselves loving cloth diapers and telling everyone about how much they loved them. I met just as many new parents who thought they ate "just fine," but once they had a baby they skipped the junk food aisle, read labels, and even invited friends over to make baby food together. These changes didn't arise from fear; they arose because they felt right. Take Nora Gainer, for example, a corporate executive who gave up drinking eight Styrofoam cups of coffee a day when she got pregnant. Two years later she and her husband started a bar and grill that serves locally grown foods.

This idea of hope also explains why one corporate daycare I worked with decided to "go green" to attract new clients during an economic downturn. It was the first daycare in the region to cloth diaper all one hundred of its children. This initiative kept two semi-trucks worth of diapers out of the landfill each year. The people who ran the daycare called it the best decision they made.

Acting green increased these people's belief in the power of green actions. Little changes led to bigger changes. Bigger changes led to new beliefs. Some parents sought out the research only after they changed their behaviours. I love research, but it doesn't always inspire change. Sometimes you just have to grope toward something that makes more sense or feels better. The information out there supports change, but we all have ideas about what needs to be done that we can act on. Research can come later. It's like jumping into a beautiful lake on a hot day. The research suggests exercise is great for your heart and pleasure is great for your brain, but that's not what propels you into the lake.

Worry Smart

Imagine an item on a store shelf with a beautiful label, a government seal of approval, and perhaps even a little slogan that says "For baby!"

Safe, right? Well, maybe.

The first thing this book will demonstrate is that just because an item is for sale in the United States or Canada, does not mean that it is safe.

Who hasn't thought, *Well, it can't be that bad or it wouldn't be allowed*? But really, how can we still think like this after the recalls of dangerous toys, headlines proclaiming "Toxic baby bottles!" and the various food scares? It's easier to believe that companies, the government, or *someone else* is watching out for us. But when it comes to consumer protection, they often aren't. We must mother ourselves.

Every time I research a new issue, I prepare myself for the horror of everything I have been doing wrong. I find this one of the hardest things to deal with as a parent. Very early on, I learned to channel this guilt into outrage: *Why on earth are we doing this to ourselves, our world, our children?* Anger, according to neuroscientists, leads to action, while sadness is more likely to lead to inaction. For me, outrage has been transformed into something positive and powerful: the belief that parents can come together to make a safer, healthier, and greener world for our children.

Biologically, moms are wired to respond to immediate, visible dangers. When I was a new mother, we didn't have a car, so I spent a lot of time on public transit. Whenever someone would shake my little girl's hand, my instincts cried "She will catch a horrible disease!" Luckily, I had done the research. I knew that her immune system would be better off without chemical hand-sanitizer on her body.

Such dilemmas are at the heart of modern-day parenting: Eat dirt at the park or stay locked in the stroller? Risk a sunburn or use sunscreens that may contain suspect ingredients? Drink questionable water from the public tap or drink purified water from a plastic bottle? Put your child in front of a video to cook dinner or eat another prepackaged meal?

Current research supports many seemingly "old-fashioned" parenting practices — more time for children to play on their own, getting them out of diapers earlier, breastfeeding — that may actually make the job of parenting easier.

When people see you doing something that may be a little different than the norm (cloth diapering, composting, asking your child's daycare to swap out the antibacterial hand soap, or any of a million other things), and they see you doing it with a smile, they will want to do it too. Really! So if you hate cloth diapering, don't do it. Yes, it is the greener choice, but greener options exist for almost everything, so start with what excites you!

And if there's one thing that my work as The Green Mama has shown me, it is that green parenting is more fun when it's shared. When new parents come together, all the hormones, hope, and habit-changing becomes palpable. Sure, no one has been sleeping well, most of the moms are sporting disheveled ponytails, and spit-up stains can be seen in odd places, but there is a feeling of magic mixed up with it all.

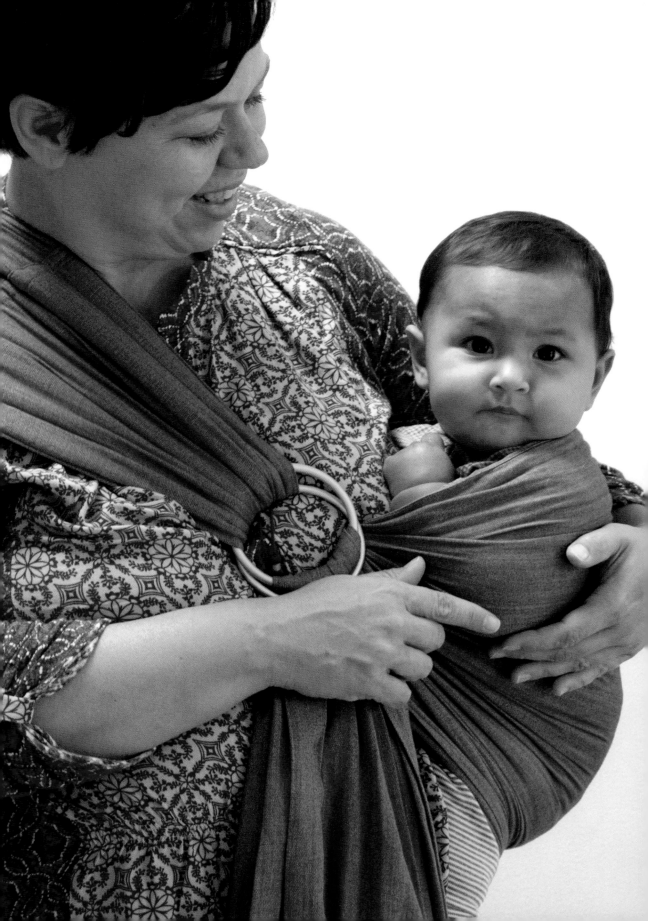

I watch new moms and dads inspire one another every day, whether it be early potty use, homemade baby food, baby-wearing, cloth diapering, DIY sunscreen, breast milk sharing, co-sleeping, or organic mattresses. Just a few years ago, these things seemed radical, but increasingly people find the commercialized "norm" unappealing. Green seems more fun and more possible, in part because it encourages community and shared experiences. So, lend a friend this book, invite your neighbour over with her kids, and visit me online.

When our green choices are writ large, the world will be a better place. Life with kids is busy and hectic and often involves cherry juice smeared on your new white blouse. So, whether you start big or start small, just start! Good research will empower you, but go easy on yourself. Laugh and shrug when you use the occasional disposable diaper or Styrofoam coffee cup. Our children don't need us to be perfect; they just need us to make an effort.

If you are looking for inspiration, check out the many Inspiring Mamas in this book who have overcome obstacles to help create greener options for their families and yours. If you, like my mother, are on public assistance, or are

— green tip —

Baby-Wearing Is Baby-Caring

Wearing your baby is something that today's hip parents have in common with yesterday's mamas. Baby-wearing can be good for the environment (saving resources by avoiding those big, fancy strollers and making it easier to use public transit, walk, and be outside). It can also be good for the baby, according to attachment parenting advocates such as Dr. William Sears, who instructs that baby-wearing can help create a healthy parent-child attachment.

I started wearing my baby because of something I read in "ethno-pediatric" anthropologist Meredith Small's book *Our Babies, Ourselves*. In it, she referred to a study in which one group of parents were asked to carry their babies (from birth) three hours more than usual and the other group carried their babies the normal amount. After 12 weeks, the two groups had only 1.7 hours a day of carrying difference, but the group of babies that were carried more cried 43 percent less in duration than the other group. Dr. Sears routinely recommends that parents wear their babies both as a prophylactic against a fussy baby and as a way of calming a fussy baby.

There are lots of fancy carriers on the market these days. They fall into four basic categories: wraps, slings, soft-structured carriers, and frame (or backpack) carriers.

just temporarily broke, check out the "When Money Matters More" sidebars. "Green" doesn't necessarily have to mean "more expensive," although it can mean spending more on one type of item (like food) and less on another (like toys). Or, if you are just ready to get started: skip everything and go straight to the "How to" sections at the end of each chapter.

Science, community, and inspiration all help us make decisions that support healthy, nurtured, and happy children. The basics are simple and time-tested. Here they are at a glance:

- **Provide clean air** in your home, even while you are pregnant (chapter 1).
- **Reduce waste** with cloth diapers or a combination of disposables and cloth, and prepare your kids for potty training from the time they are babies (chapter 2).
- **Breastfeed** if possible. If this is not possible, find healthier alternatives to conventional formulas and bottles (chapter 3).
- **Feed your family healthy food,** and get started from pre-conception (chapter 4).
- **Make your kids "edible,"** because what goes *on* the body is as important as what goes *in* it (chapter 5).
- **Take your child's play seriously,** and take it outside (chapter 6).
- **Research.** Check out the Resource List, Further Reading, and Sources to find greener parenting supplies, books of interest, and links to studies in the book that may have piqued your interest.

You can begin all these steps during pre-conception. Remember that by caring for yourself (both mother and father) during pre-conception and pregnancy, you are also caring for your child.

I could have made this book a million pages long, but new parents are busy and large books are overwhelming (and hard on your chest when you fall asleep reading them). If you have further questions, or just want to know "What next?" as your children grow up, I encourage you to visit me online at *www.thegreenmama.com*. I want to hear from you!

Brain Changer: Neuroscience for Parents

Neuroscience now tells us that our brains are more malleable than we previously understood. Our brains develop and change throughout our lives, particularly when we are young and when we become parents, and those changes may actually help make us better citizens as well as better parents.

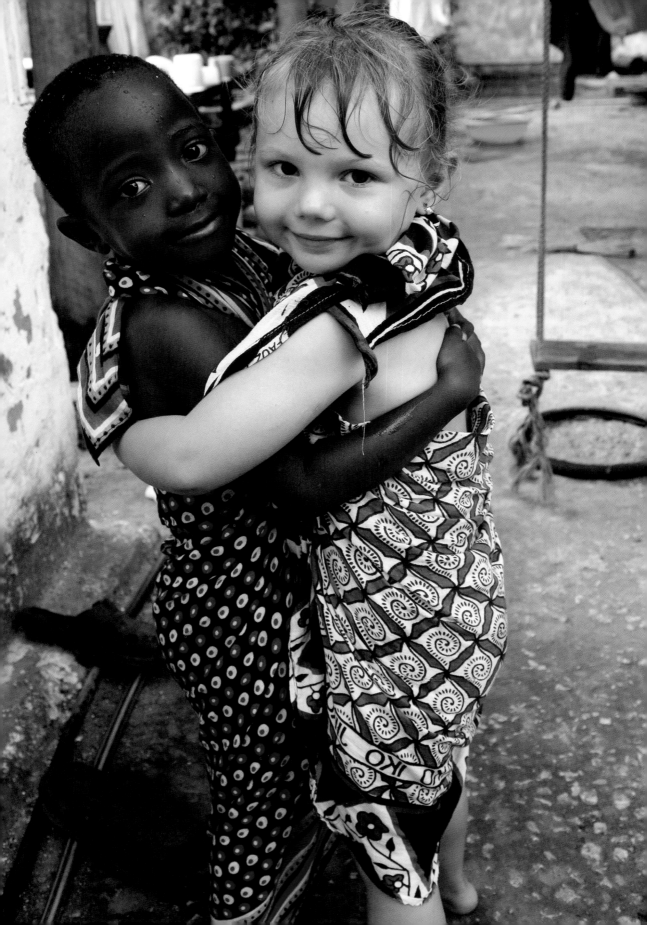

Health Trends at a Glance

Life expectancy
Canada is ranked 13th in the world at 81.5 years; the United States is 51st at just over 78.5 years.

Asthma
Rates in America and Canada have quadrupled in the last 20 years; 10 percent of children now have asthma according to 2011 numbers from the Centers for Disease Control.

Invasive cancers
Rates in children rose 29 percent in the 20 years leading up to the National Cancer Institute's most recent (2004) numbers.

Obesity
Rates have more than doubled in the past 30 years for juveniles in both the United States and Canada; nearly a third of all children in both countries are overweight or obese.

Type 2 Diabetes
The disease used to occur almost exclusively in adults, but one in three American and Canadian children born in 2000 will be diagnosed with the disease at some point.

ADHD
Reported cases rose 41 percent between 2003 and 2013; one in 10 school-aged children is now diagnosed with ADHD in the United States, with similar rates assumed for Canada.

Autism spectrum disorders
Affect one in 88 North American children; one in six American children had a developmental disability in 2006–08, according to the CDC (ranging from mild speech impairments to serious developmental disabilities such as autism).

Mental health
Mental health disorders affect 10 to 20 percent of Canadian youth; suicide accounts for 24 percent of all deaths among 15- to 24-year-olds in Canada.

Infertility
According to a 2010 survey, infertility rose from 8.5 percent in 1992 to 15 percent in 2009–10. It now affects up to 16 percent of couples in both the United States and Canada.

The infant brain is particularly malleable and produces trillions more synapses between nerve cells than adult brains. Baby's first attachments imprint his brain and shape future behaviours, so a positive first attachment with a caregiver can significantly promote future resiliency — helping the child control his impulses, emotions, and reactions — despite life's challenges. Brains change throughout a lifetime, and loving relationships continue to be profound brain changers.

And then there's the "mama brain." Personally, during pregnancy and lactation, I felt like my brains had been sucked out of my boobs, but science suggests that mothers might actually end up with extra baby smarts. Imaging of new mothers' brains shows an increase in grey matter or "new brain" in the parietal lobes and prefrontal cortex. This provides a brain boost for things such as multitasking, planning, and handling stress. Motherhood also changes a person's reaction to smells and sounds; new moms find the smell of their own baby's poo less offensive than the poo of other babies, but find the sound of their own baby crying more disturbing than the cry of someone else's.

Involved dads get smarter, too. The research, based on rodent studies, suggests that the brains of fathers can both "rewire" and develop new neurons. Dads can also get doses of prolactin (the hormone that stimulates lactation in a woman) and oxytocin, both of which are linked to positive paternal behaviours as well as with new neuron development.

Habits shape your brain. The first time you do something, a new path is laid down through the mind. The next time, the path is a bit easier to find, and so on until the path is an ingrained neural shortcut. Changing a habit means changing the brain. Luckily our brains are made extra malleable during parenthood to help make all the new habits of parenthood a little easier.

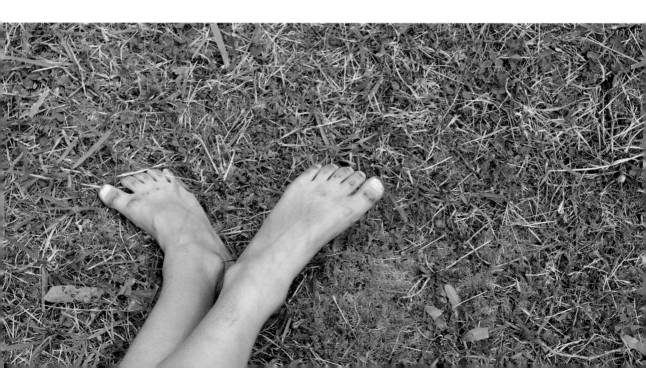

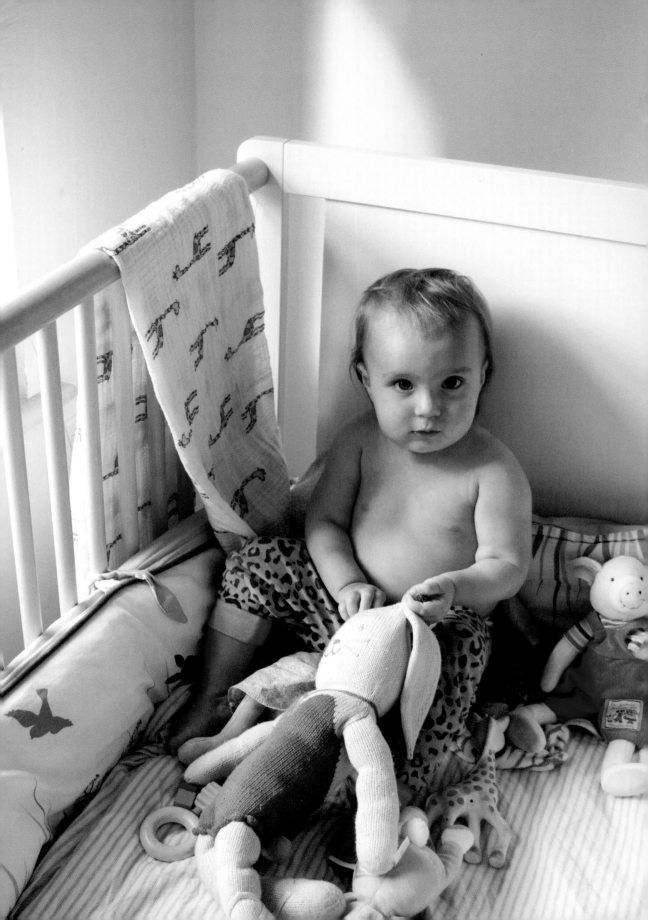

chapter one

Greening the Home and Nursery

• •

My grandma once told me a story about a Home Economics class she attended in which the students practised all sorts of things on real babies, including giving the wee ones their naps by an open window. I used to laugh at this, but now I know that opening a window or turning on a fan can improve indoor air quality and may reduce the chances of SIDS. Wherever your baby sleeps, whether in a closet or in a room of his own, let my grandma's practice help you become your own green designer.

Today, many babies sleep in what can be the most toxic room of our homes. Whether you redecorate a closet or spare room or build a new addition, those new cribs, change tables, paints, carpets, curtains, and cute little stickers used to create that special space all have the potential to off-gas (release chemicals) into the air. These chemicals can then enter the new baby's lungs. My newborn slept in the same room with me, but we made the same mistake: a bunch of new items in a tiny space with windows closed against drafts. Unfortunately, safety ratings on most of these products only address the immediate risks, like baby's head getting stuck between the bars on the crib, but not other issues that can affect your child's long-term health.

Think Like a Green Designer

When you're looking at all products, especially those for your baby, the easiest way to think like a green designer is to simply think like your grandmother would have. Ask yourself: *Will this product bring me closer to my baby or will it be just another thing to trip over at night?* When embarking on a green design project — whether home, nursery, or closet — consider the following:

- Is this new product or material really necessary, or can I do without it?
- Was there harm done to the planet or to workers when it was produced?
- How will it affect the air inside my home to use this product or material?
- What will I do with this product when I am done with it? Can it be reused easily or disposed of safely?
- Does this product have a credible green certification?

Most truly green products answer some of these questions somewhere on the label and then back up their claims with a third-party green certification like EcoLogo, Greenguard, or Green Seal. If the product isn't specific about how or why it is green or doesn't have a third-party certifier on the label, and the manufacturer or salesperson can't give you satisfactory answers, then it probably isn't a green product. (Even if it has many fancy eco-sounding words all over the package.) If the label leaves you confused, or you get a bad feeling, trust your instincts. Parents are usually better green detectives than they realize.

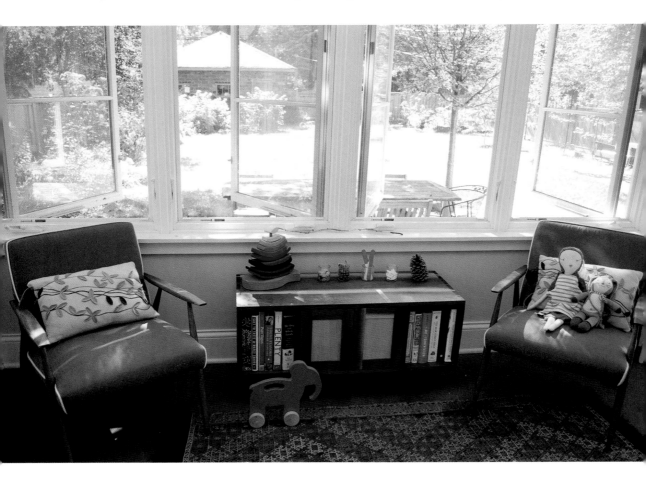

The Research

When most of us think about air pollution, what comes to mind is smokestacks that emit particulates into the air, the smog that hangs over a city, or the gunk that comes out of the tailpipes of vehicles. But indoor air pollution may pose an even greater risk to our children. The air *inside* our homes and buildings is typically two to five times more polluted than the outside air. Often it is the spaces our children frequent that are the most polluted: old school buildings, daycare spaces, and our own home nurseries. Not only are these indoor spaces more polluted, but on average our kids spend 90 percent of their time there.

Children are particularly vulnerable to problems with indoor air because they breathe 50 percent more air per pound of body weight than adults. More physical activity means they take air deeper into their developing lungs and a faster metabolism means they absorb more contaminants faster. If a child accidentally swallows something contaminated with lead, for instance, he would absorb almost half of it, while an adult who swallowed the same would only absorb about one-tenth of it. Many indoor air pollutants also settle on or near the ground, where kids can easily be exposed — by putting things in their mouths, crawling, or simply breathing. Air pollution can also accumulate in the mother's fatty tissue to be passed to the baby during pregnancy and through breastfeeding.

Children don't detoxify as well as adults do either, and a fetus can't detoxify at all. Adults store away many contaminants in our fat or excrete them. In children, this doesn't happen, so toxins have more opportunity to mess with a child's rapidly developing organ systems. Adults also rely on a blood-brain barrier to help protect their brains from many of the chemicals floating around in their bodies. Babies, however, don't fully develop that barrier until six months of age. Similarly, a baby's immune system isn't fully developed. "Everything in moderation" just doesn't apply when it comes to young children. It only takes a tiny amount of the wrong pollutant at the wrong time to profoundly impact a child's development.

Pollution in indoor air has been linked to every one of a parent's worst nightmares: stillbirths, birth defects, SIDS, lower IQs, respiratory infections, neurological disorders, hormone disruption, cancer, and other life-threatening illnesses. One of the most obvious of these illnesses is childhood asthma, which many are now considering to be at epidemic levels in North America.

Why Is Our Indoor Air So Polluted?

In most of our homes, the answer to this question is, "because we have made it that way." The pollution most often comes from things we bring into the house that release their chemical ingredients into the air of our home. Furniture, stinky cleaning supplies, paints, or any of the new baby items mentioned above are common culprits.

Pollution also gets tracked in on our shoes, sucked in the door from an attached garage, or wafts in through an air intake. Energy-efficient buildings are great in many ways, but they can keep fresh air from flowing into and through a house.

The great upside of indoor air pollution is that it can be much easier for a parent to *do something about* than outdoor air pollution. You just need to understand what is polluting your home, and then remove the sources.

To learn more about the chemicals mentioned in this chapter, including form-aldehyde, VOCs, and chemical flame retardants, please refer to Appendix 1: The ABCs of Common Household Toxins.

The following is a list of some of the most common sources of indoor air pollution:

- **Household Cleaning Products and Other Chemicals Used Indoors:** There are currently about 17,000 petrochemicals available for use in your home. These chemicals can be released into the air when used or stored improperly and are a major source of childhood poisonings.
- **Outside Pollutants:** Pesticides, heavy metals, radon, and other outdoor air pollutants can be tracked in or leak into homes. Radon is found in soil. It can't be seen, smelled, or tasted, but it is the leading cause of lung cancer among non-smokers. Heavy metals such as lead, mercury, and arsenic can end up in the soil or be found in older outdoor playgrounds and decks constructed with older pressure-treated wood, which contained arsenic compounds. These heavy metals are routinely found in household dust, in carpets, and even on toys.
- **Mould and Mildew:** If drywall, paper, or wood becomes moist and doesn't dry out within 48 hours, mould can begin to grow. Mould colonies release spores that cause allergies and respiratory problems.
- **By-Products of Combustion:** Carbon monoxide and formaldehyde can come from leaking chimneys, faulty furnaces, second-hand cigarette smoke, or automobile exhaust from an attached garage.
- **Building Materials and Furnishings:** The home's largest polluters are often the furniture and finishes, including paint, wallpaper, carpeting, furniture, pressed wood, the glues that hold down flooring and tiles, PVC products, curtains, fabric and foam in our sofas, electronics, cords, and permanent-press and fire-resistant fabrics.

What Is Polluting Your Nursery?

You don't need a fancy nursery to keep your baby safe. Indeed, both the American and Canadian pediatric associations recommend that baby sleep in your room for the first six months, but in his own crib. While the ideal solution may be for your

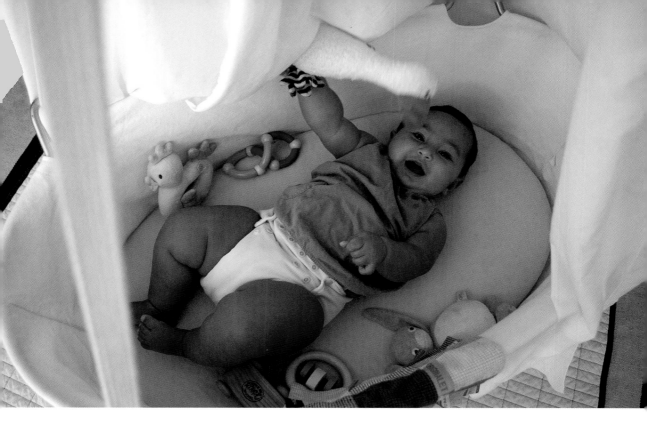

baby to have a truly organic mattress in an all-wood, naturally finished crib, he will be just fine in that handed-down bassinet with a few towels folded in the bottom and the window open, or any number of other possibilities from the "How to Green the Nursery" section at the end of this chapter.

Furniture

Furniture is the most significant source of formaldehyde exposure in your home. In a nursery it is the crib, change table, and rocking chair to eye with suspicion, but bookcases, cabinets, and other furniture found in the rest of the home may also contain formaldehyde. The VOCs may be hiding out in the material itself (particularly in composite materials such as pressed wood or particle board), in the glues that hold it together, and in the finishes.

Neither the Canadian nor the U.S. government regulates cribs for VOCs, including formaldehyde, despite increasing scientific data about their long-term health effects. Similarly, the national limits on heavy metals (which can be found in paints and finishes) in children's furniture aren't stringent enough according to many experts.

Cradles, bassinets, and co-sleepers can be affordable alternatives to buying a crib (a co-sleeper is a small crib or cradle-like structure that attaches to the parent's bed on one side). However, they can suffer from the same problems as cribs, and contain composite materials, vinyl, or flame-retardant chemical additives. Luckily, buying an all-wood, naturally finished cradle, bassinet, or co-sleeper is possible and much less expensive than buying the same in a crib.

Getting Political

Mae Burrows is the face of the new Earth Mother. As the executive director of Toxic Free! Canada, awards flew her way for groundbreaking work that brought together communities, workers, and environmentalists. She has led campaigns to save the salmon, protect workers' and individuals' rights to know about toxins in the workplace, and has produced numerous reports on toxins in various consumer products. Once people were safer in the workplace, they would ask Mae, "What do I do now at home?" It got Mae started on the campaign to get labels on products that contain suspected or known carcinogens. Industry has fought back. Companies here take the attitude of innocent until proven guilty, she says. But with few requirements for testing and the industry left to police itself, the human exposures to carcinogens are adding up. "If you tell Canadians that they don't have the right to know what's in their products, they get mad," says Mae. They may have to get a lot madder, however, to prompt change: "The market does nothing by itself. You have to get the crowd," says Mae.

Mattresses

Your baby will spend far more time sleeping — face pressed against his crib mattress and sheets — than awake. Investing in a truly green option is worth it. Be particularly vigilant for greenwashing here because the terms "organic" and "natural" are not regulated in this industry and thus can be meaningless when it comes to finding a healthy mattress. Indeed, a company can use organic cotton but still use harmful chemical flame retardants and polyurethane foam. Do your research to find out what's really inside.

Polyurethane foam makes up the majority of mattresses and is made from petroleum. It typically contains and off-gases various industrial solvents, such as toluene, benzene, and formaldehyde. Polyurethane foam is highly combustible and so it is almost always treated with a chemical flame retardant. Many of these chemical flame retardants don't stay in the mattress, couch, or change table pad. Like a wild toddler, they are hard to contain, and end up in household dust. They continue to be released throughout the life of the material. Thus, *mattresses don't get safer over time*. In fact, some studies suggest that mattresses get significantly yuckier as they age, because they can also accumulate dust mites, bacteria, and mould.

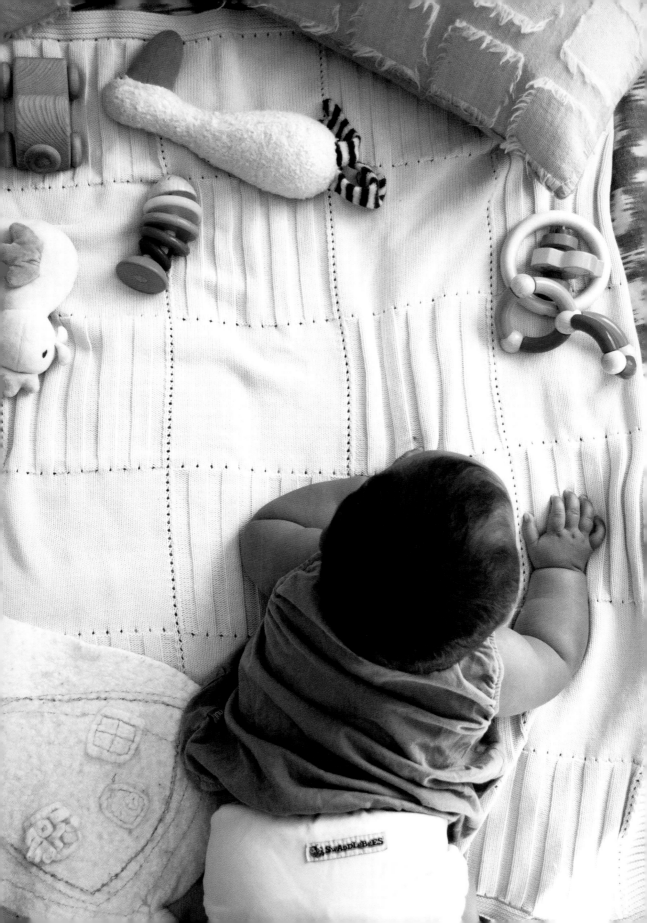

The vinyl (PVC) that encases most crib mattresses contains traces of both lead and phthalates and is considered one of the worst plastics for the environment and for children. It helps keep the inner mattress "dry" if a baby leaks, but it can also hide mould, mildew, and dust mites. I think mattresses, like buildings, are less toxic and less likely to harbour mould if they can breathe. PVC is also flammable, so chemical fire retardants, often containing traces of arsenic, antimony, and phosphorus, get applied to the mattress cover.

Be skeptical of additives that sound green, but aren't proven to be. For instance, "soy foam" is just polyurethane-based foam with a touch of soy added to make it sound greener than it is.

When Money Matters More

The last thing my mom was thinking about when she had three kids while on welfare was whether to get a natural mattress. And, when our daughter was ready for a "real kid" mattress, we couldn't afford it at the time.

So, what's affordable and does not contain foam, polyester, or vinyl?

Just about anything can work as a mattress for a little baby as long as it is firm, 100 percent cotton or pure wool (or a mix of the two), and there are no gaps for the baby to fall into along the edges. Be familiar with the best practices for preventing SIDS and add your Green Mama know-how to that.

When my youngest was a baby, she spent some time in a little cradle next to our bed, and we made her own "mattress" from layers of pure cotton towels with an organic sheet over them. It was easy to wash, firm, and fit tightly.

For an older child, things get both harder and easier. After about a year, SIDS isn't an issue anymore, but your child might start to complain about sleeping on a few folded towels. When my daughter was four, we made do for months with a couple of blow-up camping pads topped with wool blankets. Finally, we bought an organic, all-cotton futon. Futons are heavy and hard, but for a child they are an affordable alternative to a truly natural mattress. We eventually softened her bed up with a wool bed topper. By layering in this way, we slowly worked our way up to a healthy, comfortable bed without compromising quality.

Keep Nursery Toxins Out of Your Pregnancy

Do not do a DIY renovation while you are pregnant. The risks are too high: scraping lead paint, papering with VOC-laden wallcoverings, or toting in new furniture can expose your fetus to high concentrations of toxins at a time when both mother and child are exceptionally vulnerable. Instead, read about the greener alternatives listed in this chapter and get help with the riskier stuff — "Grandma, here's a ladder. Can you scrape the old paint?" Plan to leave the house for a few days after big work happens, like painting or building a new wall.

Bedding

Once you have invested in a truly natural mattress for your child, it won't seem so crazy to buy an organic cotton sheet. We've made this financial investment seem easier in our house by foregoing top sheets and just buying the fitted bottoms.

Conventional cotton is the most pesticide-intensive crop in the world, responsible for more than 10 percent of total world use (over $2.6 billion worth of pesticide!) Also, cotton is usually bleached with chlorine bleach (producing dioxins) and soaked in chemical dyes (containing heavy metals). The chemical treatments and detergent residues found on bedding are a common source of eczema rashes in babies.

Materials that are labelled "wrinkle resistant," "permanent-press," or "stain-resistant" have had a chemical finish added to them, and these finishes may contain formaldehyde (seriously, it's everywhere). Also, beware of new performance blends made from anti-microbial fabrics, flame-retardant materials, or that use fragrance encapsulating technologies. Washing may release some of these chemicals (perhaps onto your new organic sheets), but not all of them.

Again, just because a product claims to be made using a trendy new material, such as bamboo, that doesn't mean it is any safer or any greener. Bamboo, for instance, usually undergoes significant chemical processes to make it into yarn for fabric.

Finishes, paints, flooring, wall and window coverings

If you never got around to repainting the room before the baby's arrival, you can now rest contented knowing that your procrastination was actually green. Paint and finish don't just add colour to a room or a new baby crib, they can also release smelly, irritating, and toxic substances into the air. The Environmental Protection Agency (EPA) says that paints and finishes are one of the top culprits in polluting our indoor air and can continue to off-gas for years after application. The health

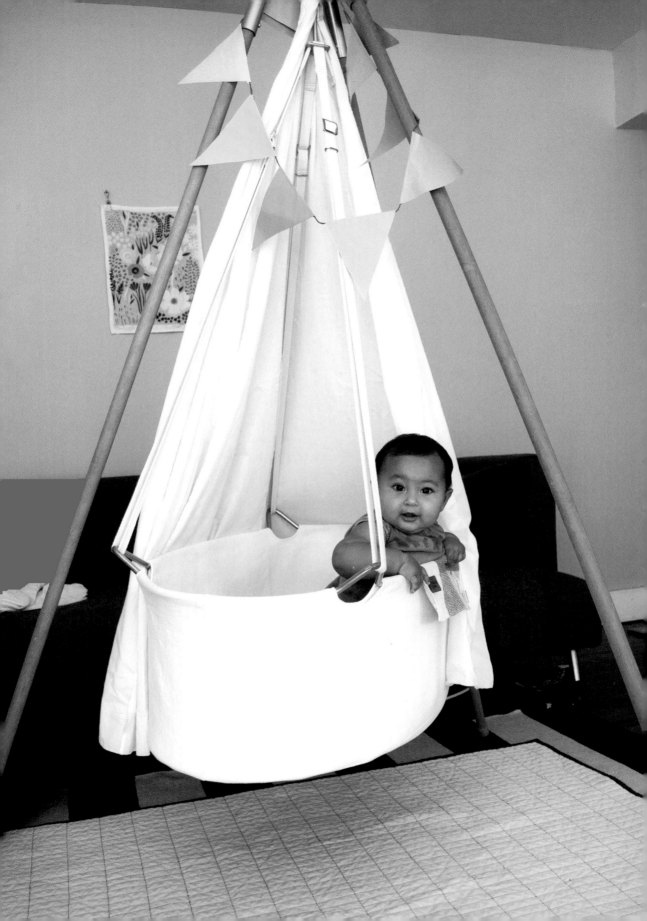

effects of VOCs range from headaches and eye irritation to damage to the kidneys, liver, and central nervous system, and cancer (with prolonged exposure).

While it may be enough to get No-VOC paints for a wall, food-grade finishes are always the best choice for furniture and toys. A clear finish may look more natural, but even those labelled "water-based" and "non-toxic" *may still be toxic*. That's because "water-based" just means it isn't petroleum-based, and "non-toxic," well, that doesn't necessarily mean anything in North America because the use of the term isn't regulated.

A simpler room, without a lot of added textiles and carpets, is likely to be greener. Carpets can off-gas like paints, with the added complication of the toxic glues (more formaldehyde!) used to hold them in place. Carpets collect allergens such as dust mites, mildew, and mould over time. They can also be a repository for PBDEs, bacteria, and heavy metals tracked from outside on shoes, stroller wheels, or feet. The greenest option for the nursery is probably whatever is on the floor now — especially if that is wood, bamboo, or some form of tile — but if you need to replace old wall-to-wall carpet, then I suggest you consider one of the many greener alternatives in the How To section.

Textiles such as permanent-press curtains and the glue used on wallcoverings are reported to be the next most significant source of formaldehyde in the average home after furniture. Curtains are also commonly treated with those nasty flame retardants. Window coverings such as blinds may be made with PVC that can break down over its lifetime and release phthalates into the dust and air of a home. If you can't make do with your old window coverings, there are a number of greener,

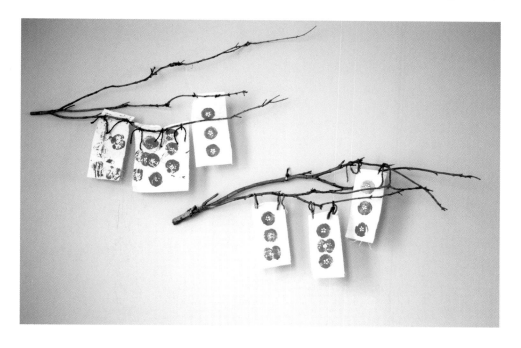

and aesthetically pleasing, alternatives. Try making your own curtains, using wooden shutters with a safe finish, or buying PVC-free blinds.

Nursing pillows, baby swings, change table pads, car seats

A 2011 Duke University-led survey of 101 commonly used baby products such as change pads, nursing pillows, and car seats, found that 80 percent contained brominated or chlorinated flame retardants and 36 percent contained Tris, another flame retardant. Anything that contains polyurethane foam, and many other fabric items made for baby, may contain chemical flame retardants. For many of these items, there are more natural alternatives: baby bouncers made from organic cotton canvas, wool change pads, and entirely natural nursing pillows. There are even car seats made using less toxic flame retardants or simply less material (therefore less to off-gas and less to put in the dump afterward). You can research the toxicity of your car seat at *HealthyStuff.org*.

You can somewhat improve the toxicity of these items by letting them off-gas outside and washing the fabric parts, but the best solution is to limit the amount of exposure. Yes, still use your car seat, but resist the temptation

— green tip —

Living with Lead Paint

If you live in an older (pre-1991) house, you can assume you have lead paint somewhere. Lead dust is the most common way that children are exposed to lead. This dust can come from chipping and peeling paint and the paint on windowsills, doorways, railings, porches, pipes, and old radiators. Any time you scrape, sand, or do a construction project in an older home, you are likely stirring up lead dust. Like any dust, this can float around the air, settle onto things, and end up on a child's hands, feet, and in their mouths.

It is important for children to wash their hands frequently (especially during that crawling, touching, and "mouthing everything" stage). You should also wet-wipe windows, doors, and floors regularly. If you can't afford to do an actual lead remediation, paint over the old paint (with your new No-VOC paint), especially where it may be peeling or chipping and around high-activity areas like window sills and door-frames. Keep in mind the precautions discussed at the beginning of this chapter with regard to airing out the room and keeping expectant mothers and young babies away at least for a few days.

Through the Looking Glass

The regulations in Canada and in the United States are often similar, but they are NOT the same. Canada prides itself in having some of the most stringent regulations on baby products in the world and it is best to remember this before crossing the border to buy baby products. My friend tried to bring a brand-new car seat into Canada (an exact make and model used in Canada, but without the Canadian National Safety Mark [NSM]). It was seized and disposed of at the border. If a car seat does not bear a Canadian NSM, it is not legal to use in Canada.

There are a number of other products regulated by the Canada Consumer Product Safety Act (CCPSA), including cribs, playpens, and strollers. These products must meet Canadian regulatory requirements, so in order to transport them across the border they need a label saying that they do so, and it must be printed on the product in both French and English.

to get your baby to sleep by putting him in the car and driving around town, then leaving him in the seat to sleep all night.

Sleepwear

Today, in both Canada and the U.S., pajamas designed to be worn by children aged nine months to fourteen years must meet flammability standards. There are three basic ways for manufacturers to comply with these standards: the pajamas must be treated with chemical flame retardants (often the case with nylon and acetate); be made from a synthetic material that has the flame retardant added to the fibre itself (common with polyester); or be made from a natural material that is inherently more flame resistant (pure wool or cotton). These natural-fibre garments must carry a label with instructions to the consumer that they be worn snug-fitting.

If you are aiming for the latter (which I highly recommend you do), then look for warning labels that state "garment must be worn snug-fitting" or "not intended for sleepwear." These rules for sleepwear are the reason why you cannot buy items labelled as nightgowns made of natural material (they aren't snug-fitting).

Green the Nursery

(and Go Beyond Child-Proofing to Greening Your Home)

• •

The following is a series of action steps listed from darkest green (biggest impact, and possibly more work) to lightest green (quick and easy) to help create a healthy nursery and home.

- Buy furniture that doesn't contain pressed wood (particle board) or other composite wood products or formaldehyde-emitting glues and finishes. Be vigilant: cribs, change tables, and kids' furniture typically are the worst offenders. Look for third-party certifying bodies to guarantee a product is what it claims, for instance, FSC certifies sustainably harvested wood and Greenguard items have safer levels of VOCs.

  A truly green crib with real wood and safe finishes can cost more than $800. If that isn't an affordable option, don't despair. Other options include opting for something smaller like a co-sleeper, cradle, or bassinet. Or buy an unfinished all-wood crib that you can finish yourself. I know families who have bought a single-size organic mattress that they put on the floor, who wrapped their own bed with rubber and a wool puddle pad and then shared it with the baby, who used a hanging cradle made from organic cotton, and who bought a tiny wooden crib with a bottom made of mesh instead of a mattress.

  If you need to green-up a less-than-perfect used crib, find an older crib (that has had more time to off-gas) but make sure it meets current safety standards. Call the manufacturer to get the current assembly instructions and to find out if there have been any recalls or parts re-issued. If there is pressed wood being used as a support under the mattress, replace it with a safer metal or all-wood option. And, remember, an old conventional mattress is not any safer than a new mattress and may actually be associated with an increased risk of SIDS.

- Get a truly natural mattress made from natural rubber, cotton, and/or wool (and without any chemical flame retardants) for your baby. Avoid waterproof coverings, especially if made from PVC. Instead, get a wool or all-cotton "puddle-pad"/mattress protector and untreated, organic cotton sheets. If your baby sleeps in a Pack 'N Play or portable crib on a regular basis, replace the typical foam and vinyl mattress with a natural alternative.

- Don't let your child routinely sleep in his car seat or baby swing. These products likely contain high levels of chemical flame retardants.
- Make your baby's room free of electromagnetic fields (EMFs), at least at night. One doctor I spoke with suggested that a child is most vulnerable to the negative effects of EMFs while sleeping. This radiation — whether from cellphones, Wi-Fi, or baby monitors — drops off significantly after about three feet. So, keep your electronic items away from the baby's crib or "trip" the breaker for your child's room at night, thereby turning off everything in that space.
- Green your other nursery furniture by considering an all-wood, safely finished, old-fashioned rocking chair, a natural bean bag chair, or a 100-percent-cotton futon couch. You can skip the change table altogether (look for ideas in the "Greening the Bum" section) or get one made from real wood and safe finishes. While older cribs, bookshelves, and change tables may get safer over time as their chemicals off-gas, this isn't true for old couches, nursing chairs, or other furniture containing foam. Skip buying items made before 2004 or labelled "TB 117 compliant" as these are both signs that they contain chemical flame retardants. You can also limit your child's exposure by ensuring there are no tears or exposed foam in the furniture you already have, not letting him routinely sleep on your old couch or upholstered chair, and always serving his meals at the table.
- Avoid wall-to-wall carpet, especially in the nursery, and instead use options such as wood, bamboo, cork, tile, carpet tiles, or Marmoleum. Use throw rugs made from natural materials that can be washed. If you do decide on wall-to-wall carpet anyway, make sure it is made of natural material, pre-off-gassed in the factory, and is adhered with formaldehyde-free glues. If you need a wood floor finish, try Tung Oil or Osmo's non-toxic floor oil. At minimum, ensure your finish is formaldehyde-free, low-VOC, and water-based.
- Avoid using stain guards on furniture, especially in the nursery, as they release potentially toxic PFCs (perfluorinated compounds). Instead, apply the safer cleaning techniques featured in the green cleaning section or try steam cleaning (without solvents) after the fact.
- If you don't have to paint the nursery, don't. If a fresh layer of paint is necessary, use no-VOC or low-VOC paints (both of which still have

VOCs, but less than regular paint). Or use paints made of natural materials, like clay or milk. Get someone else (who is not pregnant) to do the painting, and leave the windows open with fans blowing outside for as long as possible. Never put a newborn into a freshly painted room.

- If you are really pulled together and you can finish the baby's room early, consider doing an extra "off-gassing" of all the new paints, flooring, and furniture. To do this, securely shut the door to the room. (You can crank up the heat for a few days as higher temperatures encourage products to off-gas more, but beware they might escape into the rest of the house). Then, open the window and use a ventilation fan to suck all those nasty chemicals out of the house. The more time you allow between finishing the baby's room and the baby arriving, the better.

- Consider a radon test (a short-term radon detector kit is just $10–$20).

- Dispose of all toxic household items (including old appliances, batteries, paints, and toxic cleaning supplies) at an appropriate household hazardous waste facility. Often your local hardware store will take small appliances and light bulbs. Some provinces, such as British Columbia, have begun to enact extended producer responsibility programs that require companies to take back and recycle old products, so that they (instead of you) are saddled with figuring out what to do with that old baby monitor, car seat, or all that plastic packaging surrounding that tiny watch-battery.

- Do NOT smoke inside your home. Even secondhand smoke on clothing can damage a child's developing lungs. If you or another caregiver smokes, do it outside the home and change clothes frequently.

- House plants can improve indoor air quality. Some of the best include aloe, bamboo palm, spider plants, chrysanthemums, red-edged or Warneckei dracaena, and weeping figs. Plant them in terracotta instead of plastic to prevent mould growth in the soil. Beware that some household plants can be poisonous to children or household pets if ingested.

- Carbon monoxide is a by-product of combustion, so if you have an attached garage, gas or oil-fired furnace, or a fireplace, definitely get a carbon monoxide detector. If you have an attached garage, do not idle your car inside.

- Dump the air freshener. Many air fresheners contain chemicals known to cause allergies and affect hormones and reproductive development, par-ticularly in babies. Open a window or try sprinkling baking soda around

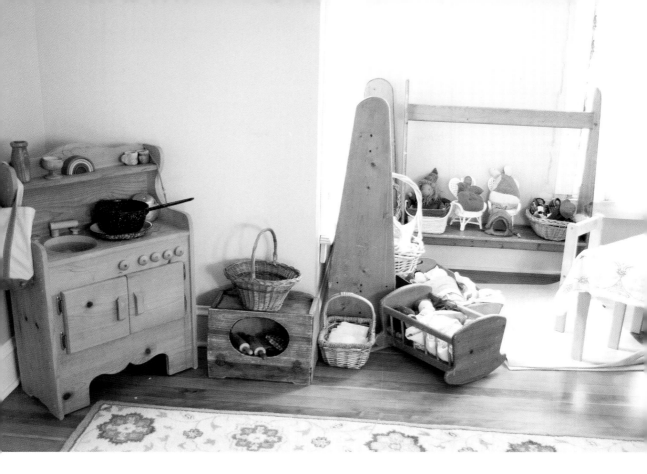

(or placing it in little dishes in stinky areas). Make use of natural herbs like rosemary, lavender, or mint. See the Green Cleaning section on the following page for more ideas.

- Choose a vaporizer rather than a humidifier if you need to add moisture to a room, such as when your child has a cold or sinus infection. Humidifiers easily breed fungi, amoebae, and bacteria and are associated with an increased risk of humidifier fever — the symptoms of which are a lot like the cold or allergy you are trying to relieve — according to the EPA. Use extreme caution when using vaporizers, though, because some can get very hot!
- Open your windows whenever possible — the outdoor air will greatly improve your indoor air quality.
- Remove your shoes at the door. They can track heavy metals, bacteria, and other pollutants into your home.
- Wash your child's hands after he plays in the park, crawls on the floor, or stands at the window. The dust found in homes can contain bits of toxic chemicals, such as BPDEs and lead. Washing a child's hand with plain old soap and water is surprisingly effective at lowering their exposure.

Green Cleaning

It's no stretch of the imagination to see how the chemicals in cleaning supplies end up in our children. One day, my two-year-old daughter decided to finish off her eggs with a little gnawing on the table. Later, she got under the table and ate a few blueberries that had fallen on the floor (at least, I hope they were blueberries!).

You may have wondered how safe it really is to dump something with WARNING! POISON written on the label down the drain or onto the floor? Well, traces of many chemicals — antibacterial products, detergents, phosphates, and disinfectants, for example — can survive multiple water treatment systems and harm both aquatic and human life. Some of these chemicals have been found at very low levels in drinking water. Even on the kitchen floor, ingredients in household cleaners can off-gas and pollute indoor air. The long list of chemicals to avoid include many that are lung irritants (ammonia, butyl glycol, chlorine bleach, and sodium hydroxide) and some suspected hormone disruptors linked to reproductive abnormalities (APEs found in some detergents and cleaners, and phthalates found in fragrances). Others produce toxins (chlorine bleach) or carcinogens (Diethanolamine/DEA, some fragrances). Almost all of these can be deadly if swallowed.

— green tip —

The Stink on Air Filters

If upon reading everything in this chapter, you are pinning your hopes on an air filter to fix your indoor air quality woes, I am here to disillusion you again. An air filter just isn't that effective. Once something yucky has gotten in your home, only clean outdoor air will get it out. If you must also have an air filter or purifier, you should know that 1) some air purifiers do more harm than good; and 2) even the good ones won't really clean the air or relieve asthma symptoms, according to the EPA.

Many air purifiers produce ozone. In the upper atmosphere ozone helps protect us from harmful rays of the sun, but when released at ground level it is an irritant that can restrict lung function and trigger asthma. Ozone in the home may react with other common household products, such as air fresheners or cleaners, to create irritants or toxins. Air filters that rely on HEPA filters are better at trapping dust, pollen, and smoke without producing harmful side effects. Avoid ionizers, electrostatic precipitators, and ozone purifiers.

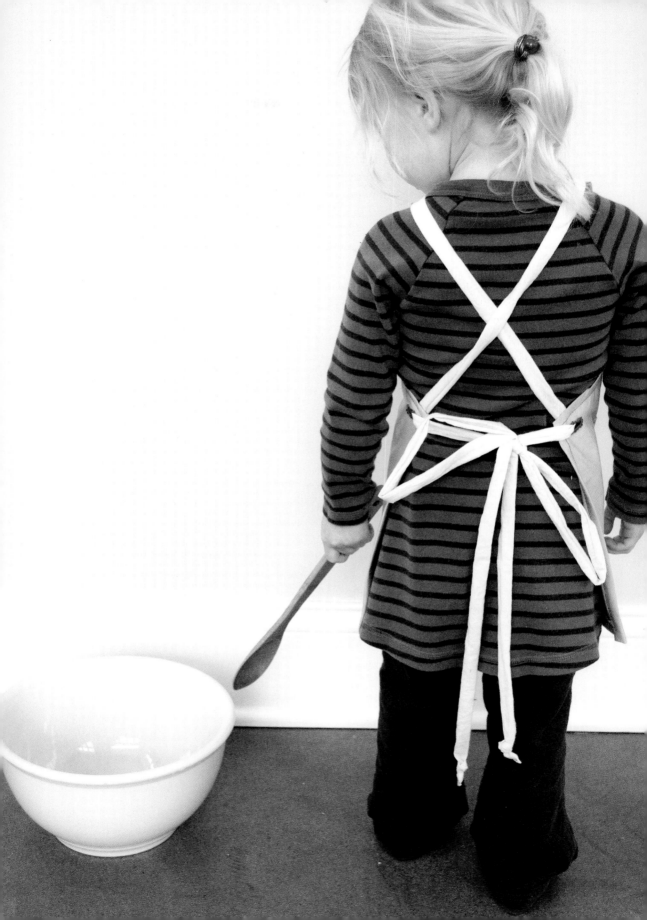

You may be surprised by some of the worst offenders. According to the EPA's "Guide to Indoor Air Quality," most store-bought air fresheners "release pollutants more or less continuously" into your home. And your multipurpose cleaner may have a little red warning label on it instructing you to wipe surfaces down with water after it's applied (otherwise you could absorb the chemicals through your skin or along with your food).

Cleaning well means using safe ingredients and ensuring they are used appropriately. Stronger in this case is not necessarily better.

Clean Your Home Safely and Effectively in Two Steps or Less

STEP 1: Clean.
Cleaning removes germs, dirt, and food debris from a surface, and all it takes is a little elbow grease, warm water, and soap. Cleaning doesn't necessary kill germs, but it removes them and thus lowers the risk of spreading infection. Bacteria and viruses can't live for long on dry surfaces with a humidity of less than 10 percent. They like moisture. (For this reason you should watch out for your kitchen sponge. Rid it of most microbes by microwaving for three minutes or boiling in a pot of water.) That flu virus, on the other hand, hanging out on a door handle, will just die on its own after two to eight hours. If you really need to disinfect, move to Step 2.

STEP 2: Disinfect.
Disinfectants kill germs on a surface. They only work if you've already removed the germ habitat with cleaning. Once this is done, use the safest, least toxic, most appropriate product. White vinegar or 3 percent hydrogen peroxide applied after cleaning and left to sit for 10 minutes will kill flu viruses and salmonella. To disinfect against E. coli and listeria, heat either vinegar or hydrogen peroxide to 55°C (130°F) and leave on for a minute. Both tea tree oil and oregano oil have also been found to contain antimicrobial properties. The sun also disinfects, so hang clothes to dry, open windows, and pull out those pillows for a little sun magic.

If you decide to buy a commercial cleaning product or disinfectant, read the label closely. Make sure the product lists all of its ingredients, has a meaningful third-party certification such as ECOLOGO or Green Seal, and is biodegradable. Do a quick scan to verify it's free of the most harmful ingredients, such as ammonia, coal tar, dyes, or fragrances (for the complete list, see Appendix 2).

DIY Green Cleaning Products

· ·

All-purpose cleaner

Mix a really gentle castile soap, like Dr. Bronner's, with warm water. Use a clean sponge, rags, or a brush, and scrub! One cup of soap in 3.8 litres (1 gallon) of water is a good concentration for walls, floors, and counters. One part castile soap to one part water in a foaming pump is perfect for washing hands.

All-purpose disinfectant

Warm white vinegar to 55°C (130°F) and put immediately in a spray bottle. If using immediately, it need only sit a minute, or if using later let it sit for 10 minutes before wiping. *(NOTE: Do not use vinegar on marble surfaces.)*

Scouring powder

Mix 1 part baking soda, 1 part salt, and 1 part borax powder in a jar: close the lid and shake. Lightly wet surface and sprinkle or use with a moist sponge or brush. Scrub and rinse.

Mirror, glass, and shiny silver faucet cleaner

Mix 2 teaspoonfuls of white vinegar with 1 litre (1 quart) water in a spray bottle. Use old newspapers to wipe the surface, as they won't streak the glass or leave lint.

Sink, bathtub, and stovetop scrub

Mix a paste of baking soda, a squirt of castile or dish soap, and a squeeze of lemon. Try for the consistency of frosting. Apply to surface and scrub with a sponge or brush.

Stain remover (for clothing or porcelain)

Sprinkle an oxygen-based powder (like OxiClean) on the stain, pour boiling water over it. Let sit for 10 minutes, then simply scrub the stain away. It works miracles!

Wall stain remover

(This one's great for when your child creates a Picasso in your hallway.)
Simply mix Dr. Bronner's or a similar mild soap with a lot of baking soda on
a wet sponge and scrub like crazy.

Air freshener

You want to get rid of odours, not mask them. Leave little bowls of baking
soda in the bathroom, clothes closet, and other offending areas. A number
of essential oils have antibacterial, antifungal, and antiviral properties — and
they smell good! Good ones to try in your cleaning recipes include: tea tree,
lavender, lemon, grapefruit, eucalyptus, peppermint, and rosemary. Fill a spray
bottle with water and a few drops of essential oil and spray in stinky places like
the bathroom, near the diaper pail, or in the closet where the hockey gear lives.

Rug deodorizer

Sprinkle baking soda on the carpet or rug. Let it sit for 30 minutes, then
vacuum up.

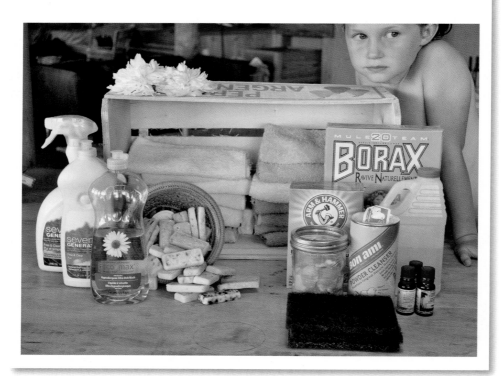

chapter two

Greening the Bum

• •

I remember the first day I saw the new cloth diapers. I was helping my friend Amy after she had her first baby, and I saw a clothesline covered with something bright and colourful. "What are those?" I asked her. When she told me they were diapers, I could hardly believe it. They were so beautiful, soft and lovely. Years later, I helped her hang those same diapers on the line — three babies and six years later they were still going strong!

When I had my first child, cloth diapers felt like the best aesthetic choice as well as the best environmental and economic one. I watched hundreds of parents make a similar decision, inspired by their friends. Many tailored their use of cloth

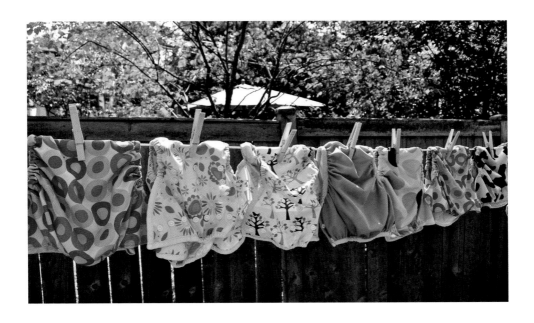

diapers to work for their lives: they would use them at home but not at daycare; during the day only, and at night they would use a chlorine-free disposable; or they would use a hybrid system like the gDiaper, which has a cloth outer and disposable (or compostable) inner.

My friend Sarah inspired me to try elimination communication (EC). At first, I thought it was crazy-talk: *What kind of mom has the time to run around after a kid with a pot?* I thought. Sarah's baby was six months old and mine was six weeks old when she called me up. "Go to the toilet right now!" she implored. She convinced me to sit on it facing backward and hold my baby facing the same way right over the bowl and to make these funny "Psst" and "Ehh, ehhh," sounds. I felt ridiculous: phone to my ear, two hands on my baby, grunting and groaning. And then it happened, and she peed right there on the toilet. I had told her it was all right to pee and she did!

I was sold.

Think Like a Guatemalan When It Comes to Bums

Spending part of the year in Guatemala with my children during the past three years has taught me just how natural things like EC are in most of the world. Cloth diapers are a huge privilege in many areas. In Guatemala, for example, they can't be found. Women use cheap rags to wrap around their babies. If they buy the low-quality, heavily perfumed disposable diapers that are available, the cost of one diaper alone is equivalent to that of a family meal. Then, they have to pay to dispose of those diapers — or burn them in the yard, or throw them beside a path. You can bet that there are no three-year-olds still wearing diapers there!

Peeing and pooping on oneself is not human nature, so there's nothing crazy about considering working with your child's natural inclination to try to get them out of diapers faster. What if cloth diapers were a luxury as they are in much of the world? It's not difficult to take the luxurious, green, and healthy route.

Whether you're talking about cloth diapering, EC, or some combination of these methods, it's just about setting up a system. When it comes to babies and diapers, there is no perfect-world scenario. No matter what you choose, including Pampers, you will see lots of poo, and the process of diapering will take time and energy. You can choose to spend that time holding your baby over a toilet, washing cloth diapers, or driving to Target to buy disposables.

For most families, a combination of cloth diapers, "greener" disposables (those without chlorine bleach and without plastic — or with minimal plastic), and EC is the best combination of manageable, cost-effective, and green. But a family's personal situation will decide how much of each one. Using one less

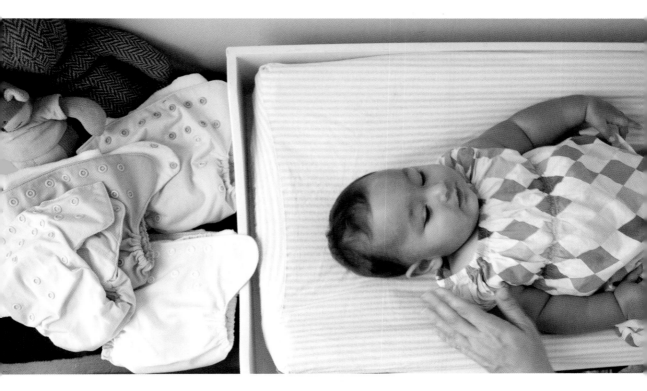

disposable diaper a day still adds up to savings: financial, environmental, and possibly even for the health of your baby. Read on to find out what your options are and what will work best for you and your family.

The Research

The average child uses more than 7,000 diapers, which means diaper choices have a big impact both on the child's health and on the planet. These impacts include: 1) making the diaper; 2) using the diaper; 3) disposing of the diaper; 4) transporting the diaper; and 5) the possibility of re-use (in the case of cloth). Also, consider the cost. Disposables cost a family roughly $800 per year (or $2,400 for three years), while cloth diapers will cost between $300 and $800 IN TOTAL. And they can be reused for many years to come, with successive children.

Diaper companies have spent millions of dollars on misleading studies and public relation campaigns to obscure the obvious greenness of cloth diapers. A 1990 Proctor & Gamble (manufacturers of Pampers) study claimed that cloth diapers use more energy than disposables. It was promptly debunked, but not before P&G spread the lie.

Butts to Bums: Eliminating the Idea of Waste

Tom Szaky, the founder of TerraCycle, aims to eliminate the idea of waste. Now active in 25 countries, with 30 brand partners, the organization is responsible for diverting 2.5 billion units of waste from landfills all over the planet. Dirty diapers, cigarette butts, and gum are Tom's most targeted waste stream. What is the answer to all the disposable diapers clogging the waste streams? What is the answer to disposable diapers filling landfills? While I think *cloth diapers*, Tom thinks *recycling disposables*. And, no, your town does not currently recycle, compost, or do anything green with your disposable diapers. Nobody in the world does ... yet. (Not even in Toronto, where you can throw them in the compost bin but they just get pulled out and sent to landfill).

Cigarette butt recycling initiatives were recently rolled out in a number of cities in Canada, and the United States is next. So, why aren't they recycling diapers? TerraCycle has the technological solution, and it isn't that expensive. "Consumers don't do enough yelling: If consumers start demanding it, then it will happen," says Nina Purewal, general manager at TerraCycle Canada. Perhaps all those crying babies can be put to use as advocates?

The most comprehensive, least biased studies, including ones from the Dutch and Canadian governments and the Women's Environmental Network (WEN) of the UK, have all found that cloth diapers are significantly better for the planet than disposable diapers. The Dutch report concluded that reusable diapers are up to seven times better for the environment. The Canadian study supported the WEN study, which concluded that disposable diapers use 20 times more raw materials, 3 times more energy, 2 times as much water, and generate 60 times more waste than cloth diapers, when looking at the complete environmental footprint (from manufacturing to disposal) of both systems. The UK re-released a study on cloth diapers, or "nappies," in 2008 that stated that under normal use (i.e., not routinely boiled, ironed, or tumbled dry) they were 40 percent better for the environment. And that's not taking into account land use differences (which are thought to be significantly in favour of cloth).

Part of diapering a baby is wiping up that cute little bum. Diaper wipes pose many of the same problems as diapers themselves: toxins, allergens, and many other chemicals hard on (or dangerous to) a baby's skin. Wipes create an enormous amount of waste: from the big plastic containers they come in, to the pollution associated with the transport of raw materials from around the world, to, finally, their fate in landfill. And, there is the expense. (See "DIY Baby Skincare Recipes" on pages 122–124 to learn how to make your own green diaper wipes.)

Problems with Disposable Diapers

Waste

In a home with one baby being diapered, disposable diapers can make up half of that entire home's waste. It is the third largest single consumer item found in landfills and accounts for about 4 percent of all solid waste. Disposable diapers dumped in landfills will never biodegrade (become soil), but it is possible that the plastics in the diaper will photo-degrade and become tiny plastic particles that can end up in water, soil, and even our bodies. It is also possible that the fecal matter can release bacteria and live viruses into the surrounding environment.

Resources

Most disposable diapers are produced using trees, plastic, chlorine bleach, and absorbent gels. Each of these elements has an environmental impact, from possible old-growth forest depletion (yes, thousand-year-old trees in Canada have been cut down to produce pulp for making diapers) to the production of dioxin, a dangerous toxin. One estimate put the resource use of disposable diapers per baby, per year at 136 kilograms (300 pounds) of wood, 22 kilograms (50 pounds) of petroleum, and 9 kilograms (20 pounds) of chlorine.

Health

Babies who use cloth diapers get fewer diaper rashes, don't need barrier creams for healthy skin, and tend to potty train earlier.

Cloth diapers usually have simple ingredients, like cotton or hemp interiors and cotton, wool, or polyester outers. Disposable diapers, on the other hand, have numerous chemical ingredients that their manufacturers are not required to disclose. These ingredients can include polyethylene film, polypropylene plastic, bleached paper pulp, petrolatum, stearyl alcohol, hot melts (glue), elastic, cellulose tissue, perfume, and SAP (an absorbent gelling material). Many of these ingredients have been linked with possible negative health effects. SAP absorbs the natural oils and moisture in a baby's developing skin and can cause skin irritation and allergic reactions.

Some studies suggest disposable diapers release VOCs, including toluene, ethylbenzene, xylene, and dipentene, all of which have been linked to negative health effects. A study published in the *Archives of Disease in Childhood* found a link between disposable diapers (with plastic) and a consistent rise in scrotum temperatures, which they believe may be linked to male infertility.

Dioxin is released into the environment whenever paper (or rayon or plastic) is bleached using chlorine (yes, as in what is done to produce disposable diapers). This bleaching process makes the diapers white, but it does not make them safer or more sanitary. Indeed, trace amounts of dioxin have been found in disposable diapers.

Diaper Rash

Diaper rash is a relatively new phenomenon, despite being common today. Before disposable diapers, only 7.1 percent of 1,505 babies studied had suffered from diaper rash. Now, studies suggest that at least half of all babies will exhibit rash at least once during their diapering years. Diaper rash is caused by many factors, including exposure to too much moisture; irritation caused by the chemicals in baby products such as diaper wipes, bum creams, or laundry detergents; yeast infections, which are particularly common if a baby has been given antibiotics; food allergies or sensitivities; and chafing from diaper bindings or tight clothing.

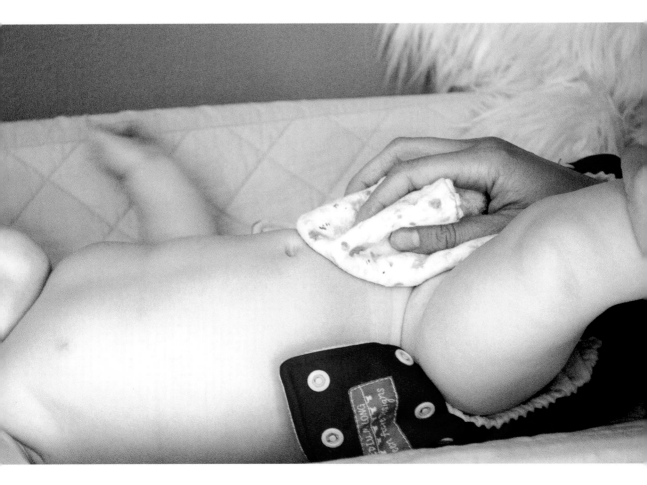

Will I Have To Touch the Poo?

A lot of parents are afraid that choosing cloth will mean they have to touch poopy diapers. Let's face it; you will touch poo no matter what you choose. However, using cloth doesn't mean you have to be any more intimate with your baby's poo than using disposable diapers. In fact, many parents who use cloth diapers and a diaper-washing service say they have the LEAST contact: someone else does the laundry, picks up the diapers dirty from your house, AND returns clean diapers to your door. Now, if only they would send someone to change the baby too!

If your child is suffering from diaper rash, let her go diaper-free as much as possible, change her diaper frequently, and eliminate all possible chemical irritants. Check and double-check your soaps, laundry detergent, bum creams, and powders. If that doesn't work, try eliminating all of these things, use an extra healing bum cream, and "strip" your cloth diapers by running them through a couple of extra rinses with vinegar or by boiling them. Once the diaper rash is gone, you can slowly add back your favourite products one by one.

Cloth Diapering 101

If you do give cloth diapering a try, you will discover that things have changed since your mother's (or grandmother's) generation. Today's cloth diapers are cute, soft, easy to use, and absorbent. Unfortunately, when you're first starting out, it can feel like learning to speak a foreign language, with talk of pocket diapers, all-in-ones, prefolds, and the merits of diaper service versus home wash.

If you are new to cloth diapers, I highly recommend you take a class so that you can feel the different kinds of diapers and learn how the maintenance varies. You can also get together with a cloth-using friend to get feedback, or consider a "sample kit," where you rent a selection of five or six different types of cloth diapers for a few months and then return them after. Most companies that sell cloth diapers do this now and it is a cost-effective way to sample many different types (see Resources List).

Cloth diapering works for most families — even for a woman I met with six children under the age of four. She was cloth diapering them all! She said it was easier because every day she had at least one full load of just diapers and she didn't have to run to the grocery store all the time to buy disposables.

This list will explain the ins and outs and the pros and cons of the most common types of cloth diapers.

- **All-In-One:** These popular diapers are what they sound like: no covers, no inners; they're all-in-one. The upside: they are easy to use, absorbent, and are usually size-adjustable. The downside: they can be bulky. The material selection varies but often features organic, all-cotton, or natural blends. Most are one-size-fits-all (with lots of snaps so you can adjust as the baby gets older). The average cost is $20–$35 each.
- **Pocket:** Also popular, these diapers can be made of a polyester, bamboo, or hemp blend, or, at the high-end, are organic and all-cotton. The major brands are either one-size-fits-all (with lots of snaps to adjust as the baby gets older) or are sized (S, M, L). Use with inserts or doublers — to make them more absorbent — that come with the diapers. No diaper covers needed. The average cost is $16–$35 each.
- **Prefold:** These are what most people think of when they think cloth diapers. Despite the name, prefolds **do** need to be folded. Most diaper services use prefolds. They are almost always made of all-cotton, and organic is available. There are two basic styles: the Chinese prefolds tend to get fluffier and bunchier than the Indian prefolds. They are available in

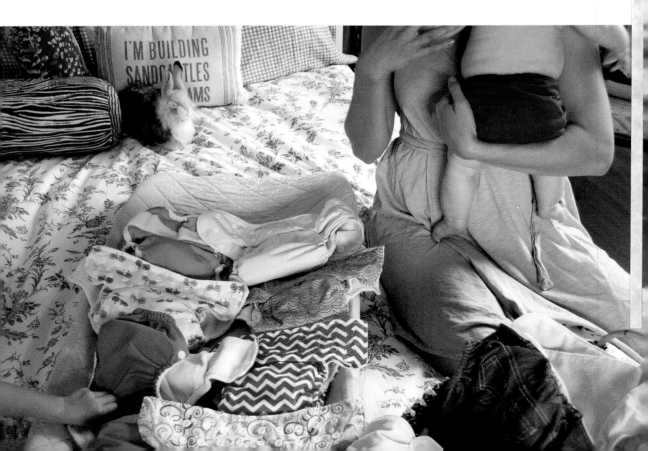

two sizes: small and large. Use with diaper covers. Pins (or their modern equivalent, Snappis) are optional. The cost is about $2–$5 each.

- **Contour/Fitted:** Contour diapers are a step up from prefolds. You don't need to do any folding, they tend to be more absorbent, and they are less bulky. Fitted diapers are similar but usually have a few additional features — like snaps — and more bulk. Contour diapers are basically one-size-fits-all (although a preemie or newborn option is available), and fitted diapers usually come in sizes XS, S, M, and L. Use with diaper covers. Pins or Snappis are optional. The cost is about $10–$15 for contours and $22–$24 for fitted.
- **Flat:** The flat diaper is almost never seen anymore in North America. It is a big piece of cotton that you fold, fold, then fold some more, and then pin and cover. One size fits all! They are used with a diaper cover and Snappis or pins. The average cost is $1 to $5 each.
- **Training Pant:** These are padded underwear for the potty-training baby. They can be found in all-cotton or even lined with a waterproof fabric like a diaper. No covers or pins. They will run you anywhere from $12 to $16 each.

But which one is right for me? is one of the most asked diapering questions. In most cases, I have found that people are happy with any of the above choices: they all do what they are supposed to do, and you and the baby will grow to like whatever style you choose.

With my first baby, I really liked the contour diaper with covers. I could reuse the covers many times and the cotton inners were easy to wash. For my second, all I wanted were the organic cotton all-in-ones. I loved them. In hindsight, I would recommend having your diapers be of a similar material, because how you care for them varies just a bit.

Polyester-blend diapers need to be washed with gentle detergent, are better off not washed with cotton things, and should never be treated with vinegar and baking soda. They dry super fast on the line.

All-cotton diapers are extremely forgiving, can be washed with nearly anything, and can more easily be stripped of detergent buildup and bacteria with the occasional hot water wash or vinegar rinse. Although I find the all-cotton diapers easier to wash, they typically take longer to dry.

Make Cloth Diapering Work for You

Cloth diapering, like just about every new aspect of parenting, can be made easier by finding a "system." Other parents are a great source of information for tips that work and for advice about what you *really* need. The following are some commonly asked questions and ideas to help get your started.

- **Where will you change your baby?** For our first baby, my husband built a beautiful wood change table and diaper storage system. By the time we had our second, that piece of furniture had been repurposed as a buffet, so we simply changed the baby on the bed. Diapers, wipes, and all the other accoutrements still need a home, and the closer to the bathroom the easier in most cases. My new favourite system is one my friend built: similar to those plastic ones that fold down from the wall in a public restroom. Only, this one is made of wood. It's convenient and hardly takes up any space.

- **Have a pail for the dirty diapers.** My friend Barry used a stainless steel compost pail for soiled diapers. We used a small garbage can with a foot pedal. I've tried a large wet bag with a zipper too. Cloth diapers aren't as stinky as disposable diapers because there aren't added chemicals and fragrances to react with the pee and poo.

- **Have a strategy for poo.** Some people use flushable liners inside the cloth diapers so the poop just falls into the toilet; others use a hose attached to the toilet to wash the poo out of the diapers. We just do it the old-fashioned way and dunk the diaper in the toilet until the poo comes off.

- **Have a strategy for bum cleaning.** Avoid chemical-laden disposable wipes. Instead, create a cleaning station wherever you change your baby. For our first, we kept a coffee carafe of warm, sudsy water on our change table and used cloth wipes. For the second, we just washed her in the bathroom sink and had clean rags piled nearby to pat her dry.

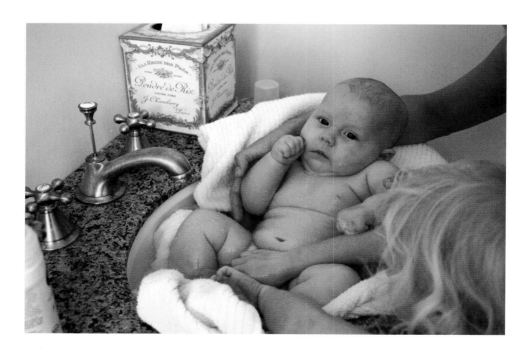

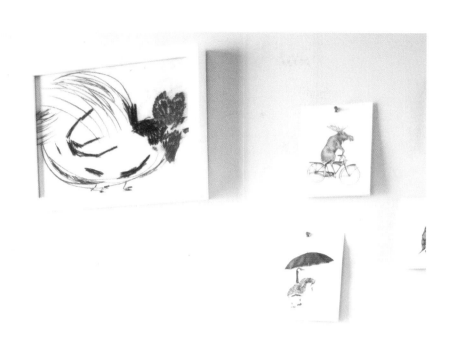

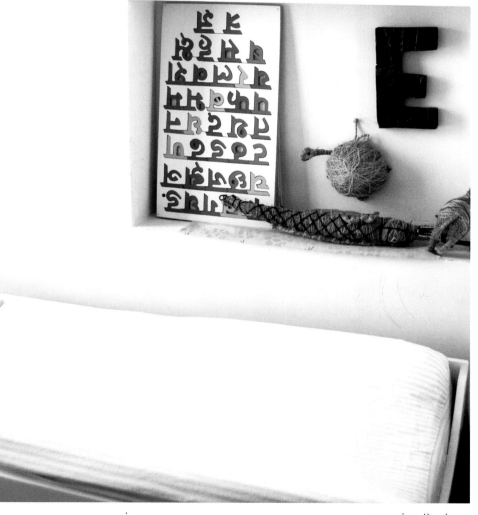

- **Have an on-the-go strategy.** Changing a cloth diaper when you're out isn't any harder than using a disposable as long as you have the right tools: wet cloth wipes in a baggy, a waterproof diaper bag for the dirty ones, and a few clean diapers. Put all of these in a bag (like a Ziploc or a wet bag made especially for the job) and you can throw it into whatever diaper bag, backpack, or purse you are using that day.

Conservation Tips: Washing Cloth Diapers at Home

A home washing system can be made to be even more conservative than a diaper service (which, because they aggregate diapers, is actually quite green already). Here are some keys to conserving resources and money when washing diapers at home:

- **Do full loads,** either by removing the poop beforehand and mixing with other clothes or doing full loads of just diapers.
- **Avoid harsh cleaners** (especially chlorine bleach and fragrances) and only use a small amount of a gentle laundry detergent to prevent stinky buildup. Consider a laundry ball, wool dryer balls, soap nuts, or one of the many cloth-diaper-specific laundry detergents. Fabric softeners and dryer sheets can ruin your cloth diapers.
- **Use cold water and line dry** as the routine (domestic hot water doesn't get hot enough to sanitize). For occasional sanitizing use a few drops of tea tree oil or some oxygen-based whitener in the wash, do a special pre-soak in boiling water, put them in the dryer on high heat, or hang them to dry in direct sunlight. Driers use a lot of energy and it is easy to toss the diapers on a line for at least part of the drying time. Less time in a tumble drier means your diapers will last longer, too.
- **Whiten diapers** by using a few drops of lemon in the wash or an oxygen-based brightener. And line dry in the sun as often as possible.
- **Consider a front-load washer** if you are in the market to buy a new one. It will greatly reduce water and energy use.

Beyond Cloth Diapering

So you're convinced that cloth diapering is the greenest choice, but the thought of it still makes you feel kind of green (the queasy kind of green, not the eco-kind)? Don't worry. There are lots of other options. There are hybrid systems (like gDiaper, GroVia, and Flip) that use a cloth outside but have an inside that can be thrown-away or, in some cases, composted or flushed. There are disposable diapers that are made mostly from compostable materials (which often need to be partially

Cloth Diapers on a Mission

Roxanne Engstrom, who is now cloth diapering her third baby, told me she had an abhorrence of the idea of cloth diapers until she saw her friend putting one on her child. "It was so cute!" she said. "I couldn't believe it was a cloth diaper. I thought they still had pins and had to be folded."

"We were in the process of planning to move to Africa to help build a school and I knew cloth would be more cost-effective." She said that, although saving money initially motivated her decision, she kept with it because it was "so easy." Roxanne told me that when she was in Africa during those years, she looked at cloth diapering as "another thing that allowed us to fit in. I would sit with other women, washing clothes by hand and hanging them to dry, and we would chat and talk about life." She said that even when she eventually got a washer, she still hung everything outside with the folks who lived near her and she engaged her children in helping hang and fold them. "My cloth diapers were very impressive to them and hung on the laundry line outside our home along with my neighbour's clothes."

disassembled in order to remove the compostable from the non-compostable). And there are disposable diapers that are chlorine-free, use less plastic, have some recycled content (or at least don't use old-growth forests), and are free of perfumes and other potentially toxic chemicals.

"Potty Training"

Even in cozy North America, exposing a baby to the idea of eliminating on a potty can be easier than a mom might think, and it can save a lot of dirty diapers, which is good for the environment as well as your pocketbook. Many parents are simply using some of the ideas of EC — regularly putting a baby over a toilet or on a potty, teaching her to make sounds to communicate the need to pee or poop, and starting the whole process earlier — along with cloth diapering to make the process of potty training proceed more smoothly and finish sooner.

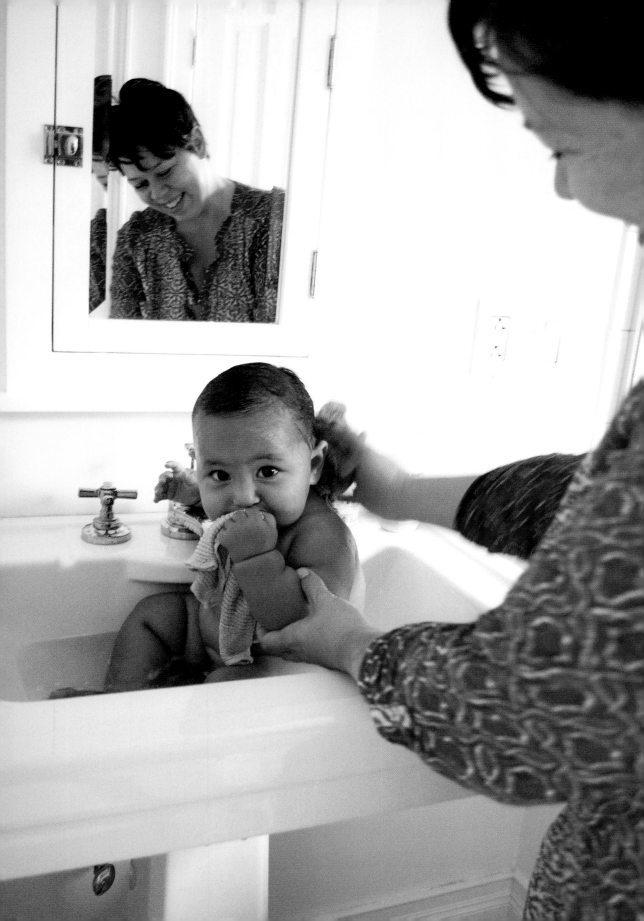

What Is EC?

EC is a process of learning to read your baby's cues to determine when he needs to go pee or poo and then putting him over some sort of potty. It also involves teaching the child to learn to communicate that "need" more effectively. This can be done by teaching the child to make *pssst* or grunting sounds, or to make a particular sign when she needs to do her business.

Most people I know who practise EC leave their child in cloth diapers and then put them on the potty either when the child makes a cue or when the parent thinks it is time (such as after waking up from a nap or every time her diaper is changed).

Most animals, including humans, instinctively don't want to eliminate near where they sleep, eat, and live. Putting babies in diapers, especially disposables, involves getting babies somewhat comfortable with this "unnatural" act. EC practitioners see themselves as simply skipping this step.

Is It Natural?

In 1957, cloth diapers were the only option available to parents, and 92 percent of children were toilet-trained by the time they were 18 months old. Today, 90 to 95 percent of babies wear disposable diapers and the average age of potty training in North America is three. Just 4 percent of two-year-olds today are fully potty trained and out of diapers.

This trend of later and later potty training might not just be bad for the environment. Research suggests that delayed potty training might lead to constipation, more frequent bladder infections, daytime incontinence in later childhood, and more difficulty potty training when the time comes.

Confused? Of course you are. For years, "progressive" doctors like Dr. Benjamin Spock and Dr. T. Berry Brazelton popularized the idea of child-centred potty training. They claimed that pushing a child to potty train could cause problems such as stool withholding, regression, or bedwetting. There are, however, no studies to back up these claims. In fact, there is research that shows the opposite.

Sphincters Have Rules Too!

In most of the studies I have read, researchers comment on how little is known about potty training and the development of urinary and rectal control. In order to pee and to poop, a child's sphincters must relax. At least one study suggests that babies have some control over these sphincters from infancy, as their bladders don't "leak" easily. This suggests that from a young age a baby is "holding" her pee and then releasing it at some point.

Urinary and bowel control usually develop following a pattern. First, bowel movements become less frequent and more regular. Next, bowel control develops, followed by bladder control by day, and finally bladder control by night. Children do not often poop while in deep sleep and most parents celebrate when, at around three months after birth, they no longer have to change baby's poopy diapers at night.

Most studies indicate that a child cannot be fully potty trained (day and night and getting on and off the potty alone) until nearly two years of age. But an understanding of sphincters suggests, and those who practise EC corroborate, that babies as young as six months can begin to hold poop and pee long enough to be put on a potty and can then learn to release their sphincters once there. Among EC users, six-month-old babies commonly poop exclusively on the potty rather than in their diapers. Similarly, by the time the babies are six months of age, parents commonly "catch" many of their pees. Children who practise EC are often completely potty-trained by the time they're 24 months old, a full year earlier than their non-EC peers.

If a baby has some sphincter control by six months, but she doesn't start potty "training" until two years later, that kid has had a lot of time to learn to be comfortable pooping in her pants. While your child is not likely to be going to the potty entirely on her own before the age of two, earlier exposure to some EC can result in cost savings, time savings, and natural resource savings.

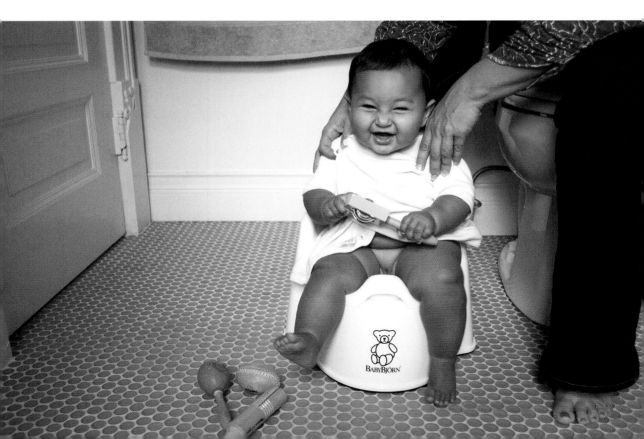

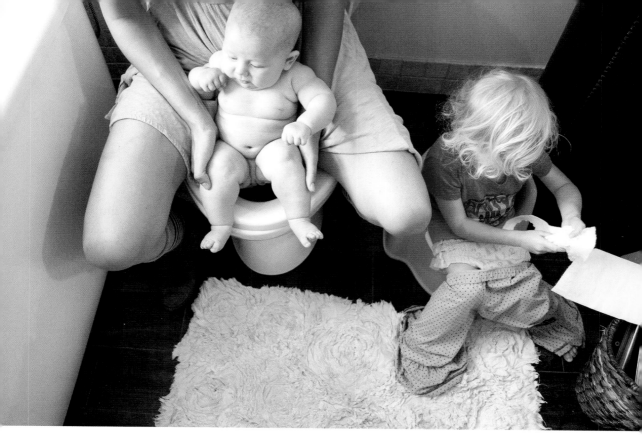

The Green Mama's EC Story

After my initial reluctance, it didn't take long before my first baby was peeing regularly in the toilet, and by the time she was six months old she almost never pooped in her diaper. It didn't feel easy to read her signals, so I made a schedule: on the potty first thing in the morning and every time I changed her diaper after that.

The down side? My baby hated to be in a dirty diaper. Other babies would sleep through a wet diaper or sit comfortably in a dirty one, but not my daughter. In the end, it seemed like it was affecting her sleep, and I took to using one of the brands of "greener" disposable diapers at night and cloth diapers and EC during the day. It worked for me, and I felt it was a workable compromise: fewer diapers overall, and just an occasional disposable.

Lest you think I am too smug, my second baby was not the EC miracle of my first. She pooped in her diaper a full year after the age at which her sister stopped. However, just as I was about to lose hope, she potty trained herself around two years of age — the same as her sister had.

Green Your Baby's Bum

(and Make Cloth Diapers and Potty Training Fun)

• •

Here are a series of action steps listed from darkest green (biggest impact, and possibly more work) to lightest green (quick and easy) to help make everything diapering and potty related greener.

- **Give EC a try.** Even if it's just putting your baby on a potty once a day and diapering the rest of the time, this method is almost guaranteed to save on overall diapers used and help you get your child using the potty on her own earlier.
- **Give cloth diapers a try.** There are many convenient systems and most will work for your family. Even if you don't always use cloth, using it some of the time can still save money and resources. There are companies that will "rent" you a package of different kinds of diapers in your baby's size so you can try out cloth diapering and figure out which system you like best. These same companies often give you a deal when buying diapers from them. There are also diaper services that provide the diapers, take the dirty ones away, wash them, and bring you back fresh diapers.

- If cloth diapers aren't for you, **consider a hybrid system** which has a disposable (chlorine and plastic-free) inner and a cloth outer. The outer diaper doesn't need to be washed very often and the inner liner can often be composted (many claim they are flushable, but my research suggests this is bad for the municipal waste water system, so it's better to throw them away, burn them [where allowed], or compost them).

- If you decide to go with disposables, it will be better for the planet and for your child to use non-bleached, non-old-growth wood, perfume-free, plastic-free disposable diapers. Finding non-bleached diapers isn't that hard in North America, and these same brands normally don't use old-growth trees and are perfume-free as well. Finding plastic-free diapers is harder, but well worth it environmentally and potentially health-wise if you can get them.

- **Find friends.** Whether you use cloth, EC, or a hybrid system, a community makes it easier and more fun. If you don't have anyone near you, find an online group so you can ask a peer what detergent is most gentle or how to get your baby back on the potty after a potty strike (yes, these are all real questions with relatively easy answers that friends can help you with).

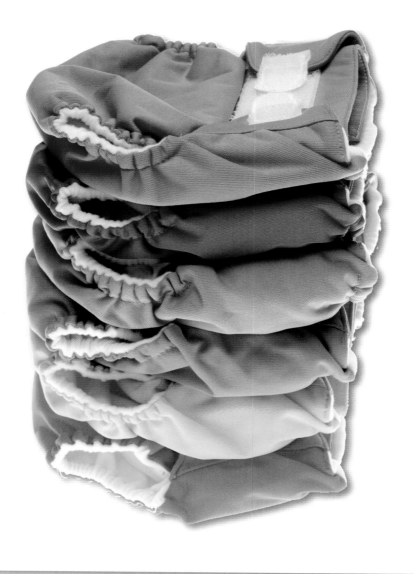

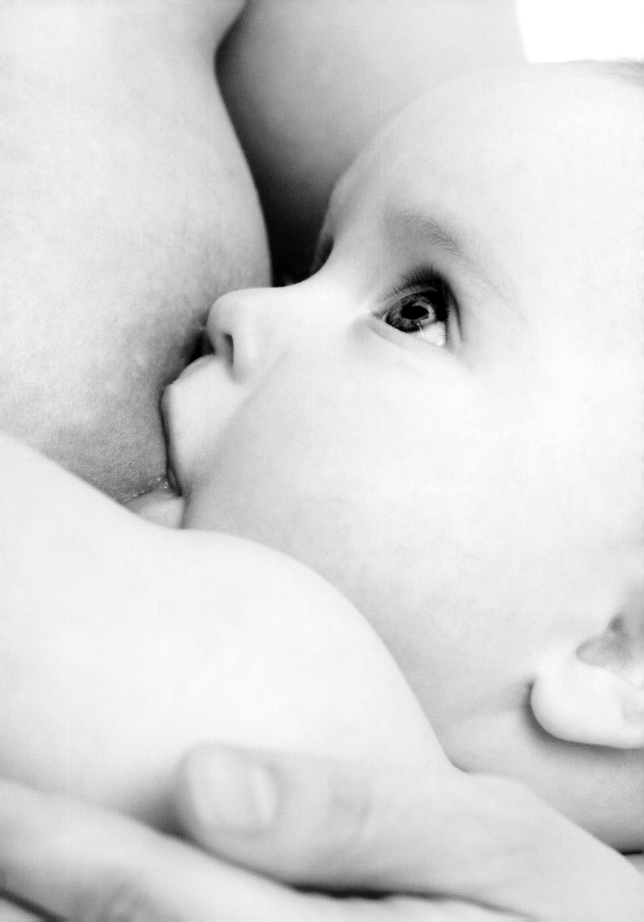

chapter three

Greening the Boobs

· ·

Women who breastfed their babies talk about it as one of most wonderful, intimate things they have ever experienced. This may be because years of harmonious snuggling stand between them and those early weeks of figuring out how to do something considered so natural that it should be simple. But I have seen more tears shed over early breastfeeding struggles than any other single parenting issue.

Consider the following experiences.

Sarah, an environmental planner and trained doula (natural birth assistant), spent six weeks with bleeding nipples before she discovered that her baby was "tongue-tied" — an easily resolved congenital anomaly that results when the frenulum (the band of tissue that connects the bottom of the tongue to the floor of the mouth) is too short and tight, causing the movement of the tongue to be restricted. Sarah went on to happily breastfeed that baby, and two others, well beyond the one-year mark.

Lisa, to her great sorrow, couldn't produce enough milk to breastfeed her first son, but later managed to successfully nurse twins.

And then there was Robyn, who consulted every expert imaginable, attached feeding tubes to her breasts, and took prescription medication to increase milk supply. She supplemented her breast milk with donor breast milk from friends.

Over the years, I have met mothers who lactated for their adopted babies, mothers who pursued infant formula companies to discover what's really in commercial formulas, and mothers who made their own infant formula, all to give their babies the best possible first nourishment.

Think Like a Breastfeeding Scandinavian

Throughout time, women have fed breast milk to their babies. It's natural. Yet, it isn't always easy, and that is especially true in today's society. I have found that most women want to breastfeed their babies. Those who can't feel awful and those who can feel undervalued and may even face discrimination. It can seem like women are shamed no matter what they choose.

As far as the science goes, breast milk is the best food for babies. It provides the most complete nutrition; a load of immune system benefits, which lowers the likelihood of disease, both early and later in life; and it is linked to healthy brain development and increased IQ.

Though all the experts agree that breast milk is best, we also know it is contaminated with environmental toxins that our bodies have accumulated over decades. For scientists, it is an indicator of how many soil, water, and air contaminants end up in our bodies.

Breastfeeding success is shaped by numerous political and societal choices. We know these impact women because we have places like Scandinavia where almost every new mother chooses and is able to breastfeed. In these countries, all advertising of formula is banned, women (and their partners) have ample and paid maternity/paternity leave, and the hospitals practise policies to ensure women get

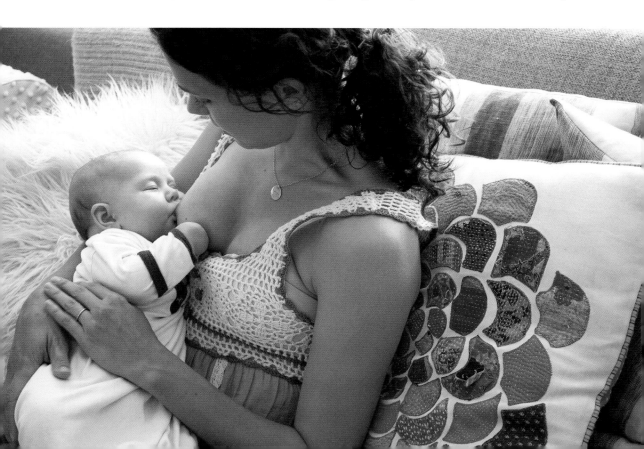

La Leche League International (LLLI)

Imagine a time when a doctor might have told a new mother that breastfeeding was unhygienic, when a nurse might administer a drug to dry-up a mother's milk without asking permission, and when none of your peers breastfed. At the LLLI Conference in 2007, founder Marian Tompson told the story of how she would hide in her bedroom to breastfeed her babies, pretending she wasn't nursing. This was the state of breastfeeding in America in 1956.

In less than one generation, breastfeeding rates had dropped from the norm to fewer than 20 percent of mothers. Seven mothers in Illinois came together at that time to try and change this culture. Together they began to compile the first medical literature about the benefits of breastfeeding and organized support groups, setting the foundation of what today is known as La Leche League International (LLLI). In 1960, the first group outside the United States formed in Quebec, Canada. Today, almost anywhere in the world, a woman can turn to LLLI for information, free help from trained volunteers, and community. It is widely considered the most influential breastfeeding organization in the world.

a good start. When high levels of toxins were found in breast milk, women in these countries demanded government regulation on industry while continuing to nurse.

Women in North America rarely have that much support, so it takes more work to prepare ourselves for success. This involves creating a community around you that may include other nursing moms (they can be more help than anything!), an informed partner (having this help significantly increases your chances of success), and a doctor who has lots of experience with breastfed babies (their growth chart is different from that of formula-fed babies). It also means having a plan if things go wrong, such as the contact information for a lactation consultant or an LLLI leader, and all the relevant information available on breast milk sharing and infant formula.

The Research

Almost 90 percent of mothers in North America want to or try to initiate breast-feeding. If it were possible to just get all of those women successfully nursing for the first six months, the human health, economic, and environmental benefits would be profound.

The science is clear. Every creditable scientific and health organization in the world, including the World Health Organization (WHO), the American Academy of Pediatrics (AAP), and the Canadian Paediatric Society (CPS), recommends that women breastfeed exclusively for the first six months and continue to do so for as long as it is mutually desirable. The WHO and CPS recommend two years or more and the AAP at least one year.

But how many babies in North America actually get the optimal amount of what all these scientific bodies agree is the healthiest food? In 2013, in the United States, 76.5 percent of mothers initiated breastfeeding according to the Centers for Disease Control and Prevention (CDC). In 2012, in Canada, 89 percent of mothers initiated breastfeeding according to Statistics Canada. However, after initiation, breastfeeding rates drop off significantly in both countries: only 16 percent in America and 26 percent in Canada make it to six months exclusively breastfeeding.

But how does North America compare to other developed countries? Not that well, according to the Breastfeeding Policy Scorecard for Developed Countries. Norway rates the highest, and Sweden is third, but Canada comes in a disappointing thirty-first, and the United States is ranked dead last at thirty-sixth.

It's not just the Scandinavian countries that do better than North America. Even countries like Slovenia and Lithuania rank substantially higher than us. These numbers aren't just a fun comparison; they are a shortcut to understanding a lot about child health, future disease rates, and economics. Norway, at the top, has an under-five mortality rate that is half that of Canada. The founders of this ratings system believe that these statistics can help demonstrate that pro-breastfeeding policies work.

Just How Big of a Deal Is Breastfeeding for Health?

Breast milk is a magic combination of fat, protein, lactose, vitamins, minerals, enzymes, probiotics designed especially for the baby gut, DHA (omega-3 fatty acids), and antibodies. The composition of your breast milk will change as your baby grows in order to provide exactly what he needs. If he gets sick, your regular contact with him will cause you to develop the antibodies needed to help him get better. Colostrum, your first milk, is so well geared for the needs of developing your baby's gut and immune system that the WHO calls it a baby's "first immunization."

As long as a woman is well-fed herself, breast milk is all a baby needs to thrive until he is ready to start adding some solid foods, somewhere between four and nine months by most reckoning. Breast milk has another amazing benefit: it changes in taste depending on what the mother eats. (Indeed, babies are even exposed to taste in the womb, where the amniotic fluid also changes based on what mom eats.)

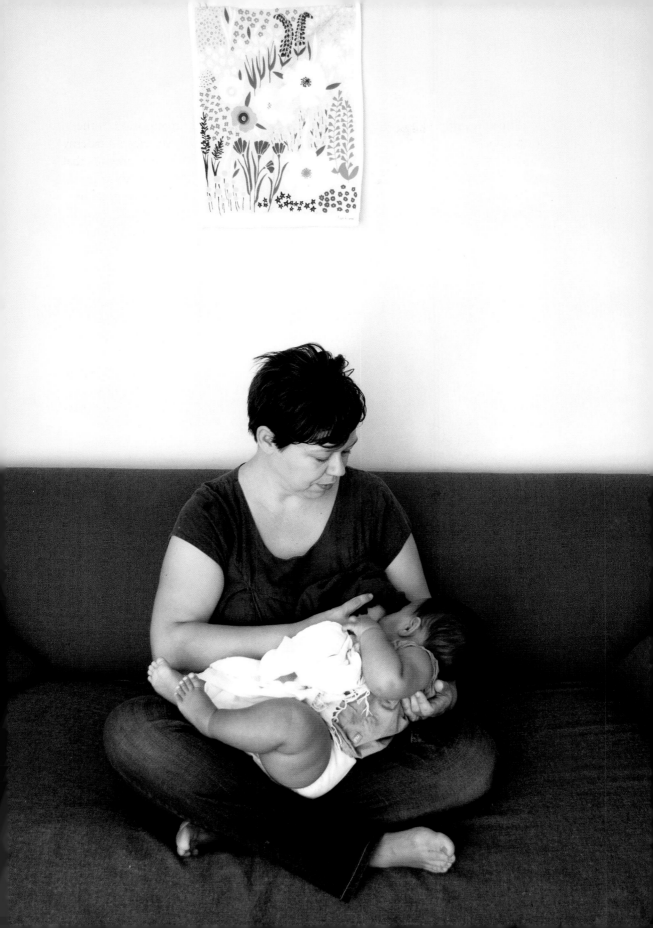

There is so much evidence as to the scientific superiority of breast milk over any other infant food that it is hard to know how to even begin to iterate it all. Two new studies crossed my desk recently. One, published in the *Journal of the American Medical Association*, corroborated the relationship between breastfeeding and IQ, with each additional month of breastfeeding associated with a direct IQ gain: breastfeeding an infant for one year was expected to increase her IQ by approximately four points. Another, published in the *British Medical Journal's Archives of Disease in Childhood*, found a link between social mobility and breastfeeding: children who are breastfed are more likely to move at least one rung up the social ladder. While these studies are interesting, even more impressive are all the proven health benefits to both mother and child:

- Lower incidence of infectious diseases in the breastfed infant, including bacterial meningitis, diarrhea, and infections of the respiratory system, ears, urinary tract, and gastrointestinal system. Breastfed infants are also less likely to develop allergies, asthma, lymphoma, leukemia, Hodgkin's disease, and both Type 1 and Type 2 diabetes.
- Fewer hospital admissions for the breastfed infant.
- Decreased incidence of SIDS.
- Lower rates of certain diseases throughout life, including allergies, celiac disease, Crohn's disease, heart disease, high blood pressure, juvenile diabetes, multiple sclerosis, and certain cancers. Also, every month a baby is breastfed is associated with a 4 percent decrease in the risk of obesity.
- For the mother, there is a decreased incidence of breast, ovarian, uterine, and thyroid cancers, osteoporosis, lupus, rheumatoid arthritis, obesity, and postpartum depression, as well as quicker, easier postpartum weight loss. For every year a woman breastfeeds, she reduces her risk of breast cancer by an average of 4.3 percent. One study even found that six years of breastfeeding (in total) could reduce breast cancer risk by 63 percent. Another study found that women with a family history of breast cancer may reduce their rate of premenopausal breast cancer by half.

Economics

In terms of family economics, the cost savings of breastfeeding are significant. The Kelly Mom website (*http://kellymom.com*) has a savings calculator that shows a family can save between $714 and $3,000 a year by breastfeeding, and these figures do not include the health savings of a baby who visits the doctor less often.

The studies that most interest me, however, show how much money breastfeeding saves at the national level, because this should be guiding public policy.

One study estimates the United States would save a minimum of $3.6 billion if breastfeeding was brought up to the levels recommended by the Surgeon General — 75 percent at birth and 50 percent at six months. Other studies suggest that the healthcare savings of increased breastfeeding for countries like Australia, and presumably Canada, would also be in the billions.

These studies look at the obvious pediatric health savings, like the $225-million cost of treating those extra respiratory viruses. None of these studies looked at the long-term savings from lower incidences of diabetes, cancer, and other diseases for which breastfeeding decreases risk. In *How Breastfeeding Boosts the National Economy*, author Olivia Campbell estimates that the United States alone could save $4 billion a year in cancer treatment costs through extended nursing periods.

Understanding the economics of breastfeeding should help North American governments make policies that support a woman's ability to breastfeed. To look back at Scandinavia for inspiration, it is clear that government policies can increase breastfeeding rates. In 1970, breastfeeding rates in Scandinavia were around the same level as those in North America. Those countries then began to implement a series of government policies — paid maternity leave, breastfeeding breaks upon return to work, baby-friendly hospital initiatives, and banned advertising of infant formula — and today Scandinavia has the highest breastfeeding rates of all the developed countries, with a full 98 percent initiating breastfeeding.

It isn't that women in these Scandinavian countries don't work outside the home, either. In Sweden, for instance, a higher percentage of women participate in the workforce than in America.

American studies also confirm the benefits of maternity leave: new mothers who were at home for three or more months had nearly double the breast-feeding rates of those who returned immediately to work. In the United States, businesses with more than 50 employees must offer women who have worked for a minimum of 1,250 hours for at least one year 12 weeks of unpaid maternity leave. Canada generally provides 15 to 50 weeks of partially paid maternity leave (maximum pay around $400/week) as long as she was employed for at least a year before the birth of the child and had worked at least 600 hours. There is significant variation in leave opportunities between Canadian provinces, though, with Quebec in particular standing out for their pro-family benefits, including a five-week, 70-percent-paid paternity leave. Paternity leave benefits are linked to positive breastfeeding outcomes. Norway, with the highest breastfeeding rates in the developed world, offers generous leave benefits for fathers.

The Baby-Friendly Hospital Initiative (BFHI)

Breastfeeding initiation is crucial to breastfeeding success, and this means everyone benefits if things go well from birth. The BFHI is a global effort to help hospitals and birth centres implement practices that protect, promote, and support breastfeeding. It was launched by WHO and UNICEF in Sweden in 1991. There are now more than 152 countries and 20,000 facilities around the world implementing the BFHI, including, of course, all 65 of Sweden's maternity centres. In Canada, only 12 hospitals or birthing centres meet the Baby-Friendly standard. In the United States, 170 hospitals do.

A Baby-Friendly institution must meet the following 10 requirements for at least 80 percent of all the women and babies it cares for:

1. Routinely communicate a written breastfeeding policy to all healthcare staff.
2. Train all healthcare staff in skills necessary to implement the breast-feeding policy.
3. Inform all pregnant women about the benefits and management of breastfeeding.
4. Help mothers initiate breastfeeding within a half hour after birth.
5. Show mothers how to breastfeed and maintain lactation even while they are separated from their infants.
6. Give newborns no food or drink other than breast milk, unless medically indicated.
7. Practise rooming-in (allowing mothers and infants to remain together 24 hours a day).
8. Encourage breastfeeding on demand.
9. Give no artificial teats or pacifiers (also called dummies or soothers) to breastfeeding infants.
10. Foster the establishment of breastfeeding support groups and refer mothers to them at discharge from the hospital or clinic.

Pediatricians in Canada advocate more action by the provinces and territories to implement the Baby-Friendly initiative. In the States, the CDC states on its website, "Hospitals can either help or hinder mothers and babies as they begin to breastfeed," and encourages hospitals to become Baby-Friendly and to stop the practice of distributing formula samples to new mothers.

Breastfeeding, with its proven health benefits and its probable economic benefits, has to compete with a baby food and infant formula market worth tens of billions of dollars. Companies spend big bucks to advertise and supply free samples. Samples go to hospitals, making it convenient for staff to feed babies formula. Baby-Friendly hospitals don't allow this practice, or the practice of giving free formula samples to women to take home from the hospital.

One study found that mothers who did not receive formula were 3.5 times more likely to be breastfeeding exclusively after two weeks. While Canadian provinces have yet to take a stand on this issue, some states, including Massachusetts and Rhode Island, have stopped or severely restricted the distribution of free infant formula samples in maternity hospitals and birth centres.

Making Your Breast Milk Even Healthier

Although breast milk is considered far superior to infant formula, there are still potential toxins that can be passed from mother to nursing baby. Yes, even nature's perfect food contains a certain amount of toxic substances. Babies are exposed to these contaminants throughout pregnancy as well. Indeed, pregnancy

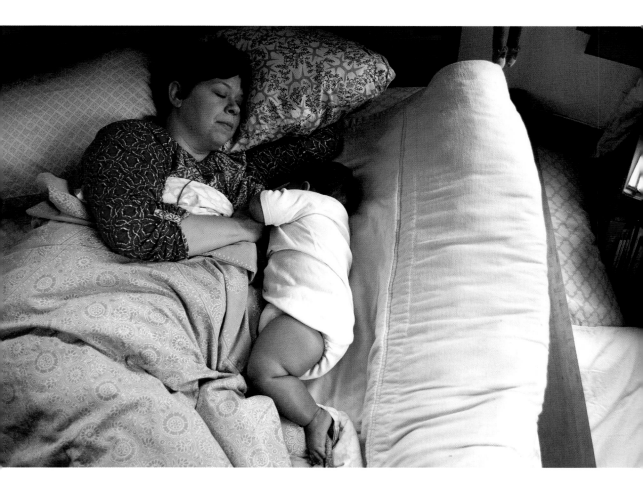

and breastfeeding are known to reduce a woman's "body burden" for many of these chemicals as they are passed from mother to child, and first-time mothers have been found to have more contaminants in their breast milk in the first few months than mothers who breastfeed for a long period of time or who are nursing subsequent children.

In Sweden, when women discovered that the levels of PBDEs (chemical flame retardants) were increasing in their breast milk, they kept breastfeeding and started a public outcry that resulted in the chemicals being banned in Sweden. PBDE levels have already declined in Swedish breast milk. Scary, though, is the fact that the highest recorded levels of PBDEs detected in breast milk to date are in the United States: 21.5 times higher than Sweden's peak. Canada's rates were also many times higher than Sweden's peak, but only about a third of the U.S. rates.

Mothers have a dilemma. All of the science tells us that the best chance your baby has is from breast milk and that only breast milk has the perfect nutrition,

— inspiring mamas —

Eats on Feets

What if you are committed to nursing and everything goes wrong? Once upon a time, you could hope to find a wet nurse, and these days you have Eats on Feets: community breast milk sharing. Shell Walker, a midwife, took a back-to-basics approach to her own childrearing. Then one day, a number of years ago, a woman from her community called her up. She was going for emergency surgery and had a baby who was just a few weeks old. The baby had been exclusively breast-fed and she did not want to feed her formula. Shell was rushing out to attend a birth, but wanted to help. She ended up putting a quick note on her Facebook page with the husband's cellphone number. A few hours later there was a page full of volunteers eager to help. Just like that, the ancient practice of "wet nursing" became modernized.

Eats on Feets provides Facebook matchmaking all over the world. Shell has also established the four pillars of how to share breast milk safely. These include: 1 — informed choice; 2 — donor screening; 3 — safe handling; and 4 — options for home pasteurization.

It can be very empowering for women to help each other in this way. As Shell says, "Women get lost if we feel like the doctors, the pharmaceutical companies, and the academics have all the answers." And what's more empowering than feeding our children from within ourselves and our communities?

antibodies, and immune support that your baby needs. Yet, this perfect food now contains some of the most persistent toxins known to man.

Infant Formula: Your Better Options

If your own or donor breast milk is not an option for your baby, and you must provide formula, I highly recommend that you make your own. You can get excellent time-tested advice and research about this from the Weston A. Price Foundation and from the book *Nourishing Traditions* by Sally Fallon. Their basic recipe includes whole milk, whey, lactose, *Bificobacgerium infantis*, cream, cod liver oil, unrefined sunflower oil, extra-virgin olive oil, coconut oil, nutritional yeast, gelatin, and acerola powder. They also have a goat milk recipe and a meat-based formula for babies who have sensitivities

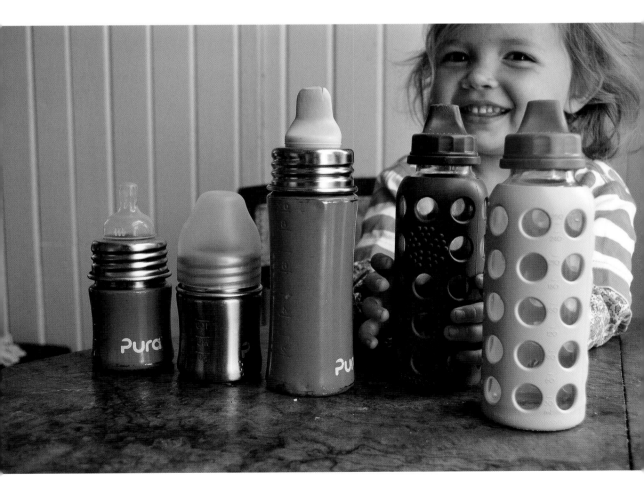

to dairy or a rare metabolic disorder causing lactose intolerance. You can also supplement your organic commercial infant formula to make it easier to digest and healthier.

If you must buy commercial infant formula, buy it powdered and organic. In North America, Baby's Only made by Nature's One seems to be the better of the options. It has a BPA-free can and was the only formula company to eliminate arsenic from rice in response to the crisis around the presence of high levels of the element. I recommend avoiding liquid formulations because the lining of infant formula cans almost always contain BPA, which leaches more readily into liquid than powder.

Also, do not buy soy formula. Mounting research indicates soy formula can harm a child's developing endocrine system and may be linked to ADHD,

When Money Matters More

Despite all the myriad of reasons that low-income families are better off breastfeeding, the barriers that they face are tremendous. As a result, significantly fewer mothers in the lowest incomes initiate breastfeeding or successfully continue to breastfeed in the United States and Canada. Should you think this is just a race or ethnicity thing, think again. Black mothers in Canada are more likely to start breastfeeding than white mothers in either country. Yet, in the United States, black women are only about half as likely to initiate breastfeeding as their Canadian counterparts, and substantially less likely than their fellow white Americans.

Why don't poor women breastfeed? you may ask. The answer is: they aren't given the support they need to do so successfully. Many low-income communities are relatively isolated from the things that make breastfeeding likely: No one else they know breastfeeds. They weren't breastfed. They didn't get assistance in the hospital. They have never met a lactation consultant, let alone considered spending money on one.

Where pro-breastfeeding public policies do exist, such as paid maternity leave in Canada, low-income women rarely meet the requirements. Some women report that American programs that assist poor families, such as Women, Infants and Children (WIC), actually encourage formula feeding, even though, by WIC's own calculations, it costs about 45 percent less to support a breastfeeding mother than a formula-feeding mother. The United States spends $578 million in federal funds every year to buy formula to feed babies.

early onset of menses, and early formation of breast tissue. It also may contain dangerous levels of aluminum and manganese. Most major health organizations in both Canada and the United States recommend against using soy formula except in the rare situation of medical necessity.

Use safe baby bottles. Glass and stainless steel are easy to maintain and free of toxins. The vast majority of plastics can leach some estrogen mimickers, especially when heated, so avoid all plastic bottles, even those labeled BPA-free. Babies can be taught to drink out of a cup from a very young age and the bottle stage can be skipped altogether when transitioning from the breast, as humans have done for most of their history.

Always use clean, filtered water. Tap water and bottled water, even in North America, can be sources of parasites and bacteria as well as other contaminants such as chlorine by-products, weed killers, pesticides, solvents, heavy metals, and nitrates from fertilizers. If filtered water isn't an option, use cold water from the tap. Let the water run for ten seconds first, to reduce exposure to things like lead from the pipes, and then boil. Exclusively breastfed babies do not need additional water supplementation.

When to Pump and Dump

My baby was just over a year old when I found myself in the emergency room for severe pain. A bicycling accident damaged my spine and nerves. I could not lift my baby or walk. When it comes to pain, I consider myself a tough cookie: I've run marathons and birthed two babies without painkillers. Yet, this pain was something else entirely. On my first emergency visit, the doctor found nothing broken so he sent me home with a prescription for narcotics and instructions to "quit breastfeeding, take the narcotics, and all will be fine." It didn't seem like very good advice at the time and it seems even less so now.

Less than a year later, I was in the hospital for the same condition. When I asked the hospital staff how to negotiate the painkillers while breastfeeding, every doctor I spoke with said, "There is no reason for you to continue breast-feeding." I had done the research, I knew this wasn't true, and I knew it wasn't their decision. What I wanted was facts. Which painkillers could I use and when? How long would it take for the painkillers to get out of my system? Did I need to pump and dump or just wait? Getting this information took a heroic amount of effort for someone hooked to a morphine drip.

Experts recommend breastfeeding in almost all situations: it is rare that the risks outweigh the benefits outside of some diseases, such as an HIV infection, and certain kinds of cancer treatments. In numerous situations, a safe path forward can be found with the help of a supportive practitioner.

Green the Boob

(and Give Your Baby the Healthiest Start)

· ·

The following is a series of action steps listed from darkest green (biggest impact, and possibly more work) to lightest green (quick and easy) to help establish breastfeeding or make the best of the other options.

- **Breast is best.** Do everything possible to breastfeed your baby. Let the cultural booby traps that make this difficult strengthen your resolve. Have friends come and help you, line up lactation consultants, and know that the LLLI offers free peer support at 1-877-4-LALECHE (1-877-452-5324) in the United States or 1-800-665-4324 in Canada. Or visit them online at *www.llli.org*.
- **Consider breast milk sharing.** If you need more milk, ask for it. If you have extra, donate it. I hate pumping, but I loved the opportunity to donate to a friend who had low production. I felt like Super Mom. It was great. EatsonFeets.org or their Facebook page can connect you.

- **Don't do any crazy detoxifying or dieting right before getting pregnant, during pregnancy, or while you are nursing.** Read Detoxify Safely on pages 80–81 for ways to gently eliminate toxins.

Drugs enter the milk indirectly through the mother's breast tissue, not from the mother's blood. Still, higher blood levels mean higher milk levels. Eventually, when the drug level begins to drop in the blood, it also drops in her milk. At that point, a nursing mother may decide to breastfeed. For short-acting drugs, such as asthma inhalers and many painkillers, this can occur just two to four hours after exposure. Waiting does not work as well for longer-acting drugs that are typically only taken once or twice a day. Blood levels of these drugs, however, are often consistently lower and may not be a problem.

In almost every drug category there are choices that are safer for breastfeeding mothers. For instance, based on current information, morphine poses less risk than Demerol; sertraline (Zoloft) has fewer side effects in baby than fluoxetine (Prozac); and ibuprofen is considered better than acetaminophen. Some drugs,

- **Eat nutrient-rich organic whole foods** during pregnancy and after your baby is born, whether or not you are nursing. Even if you are the dad, those first few months after having a baby are physically intense for all involved, so choose foods that support a sustained energy level. Nursing mothers need even more calories than pregnant moms — about 800 extra calories a day.
- **Nurture all involved.** Some consider the first three months to be the "fourth trimester." Keep your baby close, swaddled, and in a peaceful ambience. Treat yourselves with the same special kindness as when you were pregnant.
- **Dad's can nurse babies too!** At least the skin contact, eye-gazing, and general sweet attention part so important to future development. Don't prop the bottle up and leave a young baby to feed on his own. Make eating communal right from the beginning. Dads, or supportive partners of any gender, are crucial to a mom's breastfeeding success: women with supportive partners are twice as likely to succeed in breastfeeding.
- **Garner support.** Share with your partner, family, and friends the reasons for your choices and ask for their support. This is key to a positive breastfeeding experience. Even if you aren't breastfeeding, you will need a community to support you in finding healthier options, whether that's better commercial formula, making your own, or breast milk sharing.

such as some cold medicines and the natural sleep aid melatonin, interfere with milk supply and should be avoided.

As one would imagine, more caution needs to be taken with newborns, with their undeveloped digestive and detoxification systems.

In most situations, it isn't necessary to pump and dump. If, like me, you are in a situation where you need to pump for relief or to maintain supply while taking high doses of a medication, then dump it out.

Mothers should not smoke, of course, but when they do, current advice in North America is that breastfeeding may actually mitigate some of the harmful effects on the child. Similarly, alcohol passes freely into breast milk, but mothers who drink are still encouraged to breastfeed, although they should wait until the alcohol clears from the system. As one lactation consultant put it, "As you sober up, your milk sobers up." Alcohol does not accumulate in breast milk. Mothers are encouraged to breastfeed on most prescription drugs and can even nurse after taking certain street drugs. Learn more about the safety of specific drugs at Motherisk, the U.S. National Library of Medicine's LactMed website, or Dr. Hale's InfantRisk website. (See Further Reading section for contact information.)

Detoxify Safely While Pregnant or Breastfeeding

Margaret Floyd Barry is the author of the Eat Naked books and a nutritional consultant. She explains that there are two parts to detoxifying: cleaning house at a cellular level and drainage to make sure the toxins have an easy exit. This second part is essential and often forgotten in a person's enthusiasm to get clean.

"What you don't want to do is mobilize those cellular toxins without them having an easy exit," Barry says. If that happens, those mobilized toxins will go straight into your breast milk.

During pregnancy, and for the first three months postpartum, "detoxifying" should be no more than deep breathing, staying hydrated, some gentle skin brushing, possibly massages, and walking as much as possible. It's also the time for full-fat animal foods. After the first three months, however, a breastfeeding woman can do a bit more to detoxify by focusing on creating those easy exits:

- **Ensure you're well hydrated.** Urine is a key eliminative vehicle, and during breastfeeding women lose liquid through their breast milk. If you only do one thing, do this.
- **Make sure you're digesting and eliminating well.** Yes, that means pooping at least once daily. Beets help the gallbladder, which plays a key role in elimination. Try pickled beets with your dinner, beet kvass, cooked beets, beet juice, or raw beets with apple cider vinegar. Also good for the gallbladder is a teaspoon or two of apple cider vinegar in warm water before meals. If these don't work, call your natural practitioner for help.
- **Keep your skin clear.** The skin is a major detoxifying organ, and lots of stuff leaves the body via sweat: try moderate exercise or a hot Epsom salt bath, but take it easy on the saunas and hot tubs, which can get too many toxins moving.
- **Keep your lymph moving.** This can be done through movement, particularly bouncing movements.
- **Breathe deeply.** This will help stimulate the detoxification of the lungs. During meditation, yoga, and exercise is a great time to do this.
- **Try oil pulling.** This refers to an ancient Ayurvedic technique of rinsing your mouth with an edible oil to pull out bacteria and toxins, which you spit into the garbage after.

Best for Babes

Danielle Rigg had her baby on Long Island, New York, at a time when breastfeeding rates were at their lowest. "I didn't know anyone who had breastfed, none of my family [had] breastfed for generations, yet I wanted to breastfeed my baby," says Danielle.

Despite her enthusiasm, everything went wrong: the hospital had no lactation consultant, her baby was large, and her nipples cracked and bled. She finally hired her own lactation consultant, who helped her to nurse successfully and discover her calling. Her first success: her best friend Bettina Forbes, who gave birth to her first baby just six weeks later.

Danielle got trained as a lactation consultant and hung her shingle up, but she felt frustrated by the lack of support for breastfeeding. She would sweat and cry along with new mothers to get their babies breastfeeding again and then the next day the mother would get bad advice from her doctor and they'd have to start over again.

Danielle wanted to do more, something big. "Why is there no cause for breastfeeding?" she wondered. Thanks to Danielle and Bettina, now there is.

Best for Babes uses the same model as organizations that fight breast cancer and heart disease. It brings together corporations, nonprofits, and consumers. You can run/walk/exercise for the cause of breastfeeding, you can read about the Booby Traps online, and you can see photos of famous moms breastfeeding and hear their stories. You can even get little cards to give to nursing moms that say "Thank you for breastfeeding! We're cheering you on, Babe!" They aim to remove all guilt from the decision to breastfeed: "We change cultures, not moms."

- **Alter your diet.** Include more nutrient-dense, whole, and organic foods. This will reduce the number of toxins you're taking in.

When to Wean?

Physiologically, it seems that babies are designed to wean between 2.5 and seven years of age, according to research done by anthropologist Dr. Katherine Dettwyler. Most animals have an age of natural weaning. Comparing humans to our closest animal counterparts on a number of life-history variables (gestation, birth weight, age at eruption of teeth) gives us an idea of when humans would "naturally" wean without any cultural influence.

If you are breastfeeding a toddler, rest assured that your breast milk is still providing him with protein, minerals, vitamins, and more fat than ever: all in concentrated form. It is calculated that a toddler getting 450 millilitres (15 ounces) of breast milk a day is provided with about a third of his daily needs of energy, protein, and calcium; two thirds of his needed Vitamin A, Vitamin C, and folate; and almost his entire needed amount of Vitamin B12. Studies also show that the longer a child breastfeeds, the greater the associated health and IQ benefits.

Baby's First Foods

At some time between five and nine months your baby will be ready for his first foods. He may or may not have teeth, but he will sit up on his own and reach for your spoon. At first, food is just about experimentation: new tastes, textures, and self-sufficiency. His eating habits start here, so make sure you provide him with organic, whole, and unprocessed foods. Let traditional food wisdom, now backed by science, guide you.

First foods don't need to be boring, but they should be real. Children are not inherently picky eaters, although some children do have more difficulty becoming good eaters than others. Nina Planck, a food writer and farmers' market entrepreneur, has researched the subject and says that babies choose the foods they need and naturally eat a varied diet if they are not distracted by processed or junk foods. Her list of "foolproof" first animal-based foods includes beef, lamb, chicken, haddock, cod liver oil, liver, bone marrow, bone jelly, bone broth, poached eggs, and runny egg yolks. For vegetables, she suggests trying raw coconut and avocado, raw and cooked apples, bananas, carrots, cabbage, and peas. Steamed foods can include beets, cauliflower, cabbage, spinach, and potatoes. Use butter and salt. Give the baby filtered water, whole milk, cultured milk, yogourt, and kefir to drink.

Grains are not an appropriate first food. That includes rice cereal, baby teething biscuits, and crackers. This may seem shocking because baby food companies have spent a lot of money convincing mothers and doctors that grains are the perfect first food. They are not. They have little nutrition, train babies to like sweet and starchy foods, and are hard for them to digest. A newborn's pancreas is not fully developed, so he is not producing as much digestive enzyme as an older child. Enzymes in breast milk and your baby's saliva help make up the difference. It can take up to two years for a child to be producing enough amylase — the major carbohydrate-digesting enzyme — to properly digest grains. When your child has molars, he's ready for grains. Improperly digested starches create inflammation in the body, which can give rise to food allergies or sensitivities. Grains can also block the absorption of iron. When you are ready to feed a child grains, soak them in yogourt or buttermilk to help "predigest" them.

Babies like interesting food. Bland, boring baby food is an American phenomenon not shared by most of the world. "Spice up" your baby's meal with seasoned broth, butter, olive oil, coconut oil, sea salt, or cheese. All of these foods have important nutrients and are good for your baby.

Let your child handle his own food. Give him a carrot or a large, cooked chicken bone to gnaw on. Put down small bites of avocado, blueberry, steamed apple, or whatever, and let your baby navigate the food into his mouth. Find advice and community by doing an online search for "baby-led weaning."

Babies *develop* taste; if you feed him sweet things all the time he will develop the taste for sweet things. Commercial baby food is made sweet, because babies like sweet. Everybody likes sweet. If you want your child to "like" other flavours, such as sour, bitter, and pungent, you must introduce them early and between seven and 12 times.

Evidence suggests that most *real* foods, including sprouted nuts, fish, and whole dairy don't cause allergies. Soy, corn, gluten, and sugar can lead to allergies because they are hard for babies to digest.

Be wary of supplements that can be hard for a baby to absorb, such as inorganic iron. "Fix" the baby's diet with added iron-rich foods, such as liver, egg yolk, or beans. Cod liver oil will increase the Vitamin D in your breast milk or in your older baby's diet.

— green tip —

Don't Be a "Sucker": Get a Greener Pacifier

Don't give a baby a pacifier until breastfeeding is well established. A couple of weeks after birth, the sucking reflex can be soothing and babies that use pacifiers have a decreased chance of SIDS. My eldest used her pacifier as if it were the sole thing keeping her from flying off the handle for four years while I studied every method possible to get her out of the habit. (In the end I progressively snipped the tip of the pacifier.) My second child, I was relieved to note, never took a pacifier at all.

Do not get a plastic pacifier. Almost all of them leach a small amount of estrogen mimicker. Your child will suck and chew and mouth that pacifier for hours and hours. The little silicone ones are made from a more stable plastic than the others, but even silicone is a plastic. Your best bet is to find a natural rubber pacifier, such as those made by Natursutten, Ecopacifier, Hevea, or Ummy.

Beware of processed baby food! It's a relatively recent invention with a BIG advertising budget. If you need it in a pinch, read the labels carefully. Always buy organic and never buy it with added sugar. Baby foods in jars, plastic, and squeeze pouches often have food preservatives and even traces of BPA from the packaging. Frozen baby foods can be a better option, with more nutrients and fewer preservatives, but even better options include fresh avocado, cooked sweet potato, or frozen peas, which can also be quickly grabbed for convenience.

Do not give in to the temptation of biscuits, bars, or crackers in lieu of real food. Whether you are trying to buy a few minutes of peace while you run an errand, are worried that he must be starving because he hardly ate dinner, or are just reaching for an easy snack, these quick fixes can turn into a serious junk food habit. If children know that a processed, and often sugary, substitute is likely, they will figure out a way to get it. My second was not the easiest eater. For a while, when she was three years old, whenever she saw cooked kale on her plate (which was often), she would toss it on the floor. One day she decided to up the game by throwing the plate as well. She cried, whined, and pleaded for "something else" because "I don't like it!"

Well, she went to bed hungry, but she has never thrown her plate since — and now she loves kale (or, at least, she eats it).

A baby throwing food could be just experimentation, but it's probably a sign that he's done eating. It doesn't mean that you need to give him a cracker or a sugary yogourt instead.

When strategizing about how to get my kids to be good eaters, I think back in time for guidance. Both of my great-grandmothers had lots of kids, numerous household responsibilities, and planted their own gardens. They would never have considered making separate meals for their children, no matter how much a child whined. As you will see in the next chapter, traditional wisdom can also help you figure out which foods are "real," why to be skeptical of marketing claims, and generally how to go about providing the healthiest nourishment for the entire family.

chapter four

Greening Food

· ·

Food today just seems more complicated than ever before. My grandma has stories of what food was like in their house when she was a child. Her mom would put out a meal of fresh-baked bread, vegetables, and eggs or meat (if they had it). They grew most of what they ate, and occasional treats of cream or meat came from her father's congregation. Meals were simple, and just about everything was local and free of pesticides because that's just the way food was back then. Kids ate what was served or they went hungry. No one snacked. No one had heard of prepackaged food, and my grandmother never tried soda, pizza, or McDonald's. Nobody knew a thing about nutrition, but somehow kids grew, children were rarely overweight, schoolteachers were blissfully ignorant of food allergies, and children didn't have Type 2 diabetes.

Food is important: You are what you eat, and all of that. But how can we know what good food is, what with all the talk about genetically modified foods and cloned animal products, not to mention reports of contaminated food imports, high pesticide use, poor soil quality, contaminated water, and loss of nutrients in fruits and vegetables. The list just goes on.

And then there are the direct health concerns for our kids. In one generation, the rate of overweight and obese kids has doubled. If these trends continue, our children's generation will have a 70 percent overweight/obesity rate, putting them at an increased risk of heart disease, cancer, strokes, and Type 2 diabetes. Cases of significant food allergies are also on the rise, and now affect one out of every 13 children in North America.

With all these serious issues to think about, it's no surprise that parents' angst about food is also rising.

Mothers today are more educated and more interested in healthy eating than my great-grandmother, but they have a lot more obstacles in their way and not much support. Many doctors have little training in basic nutrition and the media's erratic health coverage sows confusion in many consumers.

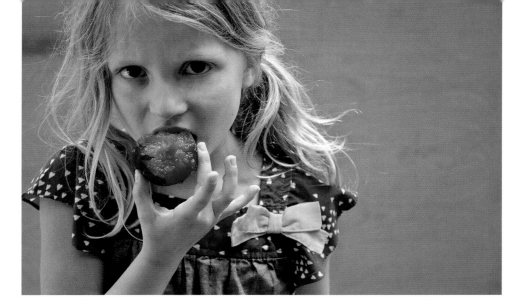

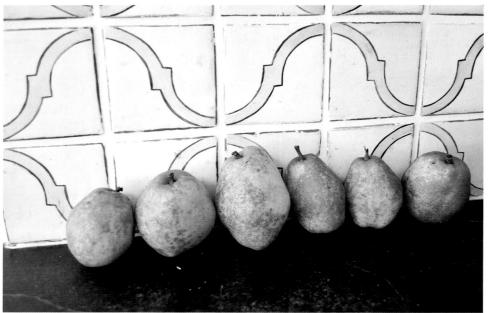

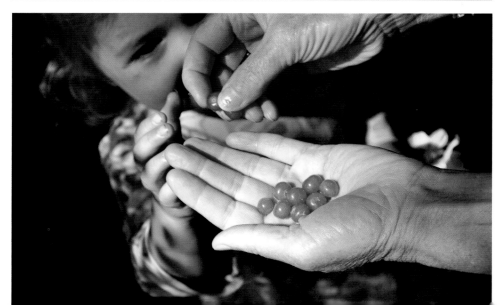

I know as well as anyone how complicated the food thing can be. I spent my early childhood years on welfare. As hard as it may seem to me to get the food thing right now, it is far more complicated trying to do it when your staples come from subsidies. I remember our weekly food box contained low-fat milk, a block of cheese "product," and peanut butter with added hydrogenated oils and sugar. I entered adulthood with my cooking experiences limited mostly to macaroni and cheese and weird low-fat cookies. That situation did not prepare me to navigate healthy eating in a culture that doesn't place a lot of value on home-cooked meals made from fresh foods. There is, however, a growing movement of "foodies," and they are spreading the joy of eating healthy, local, and organic.

Think Like Your Great-Grandmother When It Comes to Food

Parents shape their children's appetites, and the foods your children eat will, literally, shape their health. Though it seems complicated, leading food thinkers like Michael Pollan remind us that eating well boils down to a handful of simple principles.

Eat real food. That means food in its whole, unprocessed, and unpackaged state; food that your (or someone's) grandma ate when she was little, like eggs, butter, greens, beans, and apples.

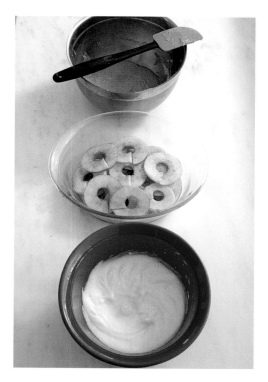

Don't be tricked. Your great grandma wasn't serving "healthy" convenience foods like yogourt in a tube, instant breakfasts, or flavoured milk. In my family, everything that falls outside of the "real food" category is considered a special treat and not for daily consumption. That includes all juices (even when organic and without added sugar) and any beverage other than filtered water or whole milk.

Serve your kids more vegetables, and in a wide variety. They will be full and they will have consumed a healthy amount of calories if you get them to eat the fat, vegetables, and grains required. Parents often assume that "five servings of fruits and vegetables" a day means that kids can get by with eating just fruit. Humans need the nutrients from a variety of vegetables, however, and these should be the basis of your child's diet — and yours too!

I also suggest eating quality meat, but not a lot of it. There isn't an inherent need to eat meat that trumps the health hazards of eating animal products that contain concentrated levels of pesticides, artificial growth hormones, or other artificial additives. Traditional diets are the healthiest, in part because they rely on less meat, though, according to food guru Michael Pollan, there is no added health benefit to being strictly vegetarian. Bone broths, wild-caught fish, and organic meat raised traditionally (think: grass, insects, and sunshine) can be important parts of a healthy diet. Yes, it can cost more to buy meat raised this way, but a study by Consumer Reports shows that often the difference is minimal — pennies per pound — and that the vast majority of consumers are willing to pay this difference. Most families can still save money by buying less meat but ensuring that meat is high-quality.

Eat organic foods whenever possible. Organic growers cultivate healthy soil, which is the basis of nutrient-rich food. The freshest, most nutritious food comes from places where it is possible to talk to the farmer, such as at your local farmer's market, or in your own backyard. Growing your own food — even if it's just a few herbs on a window sill — has the added benefit of help-

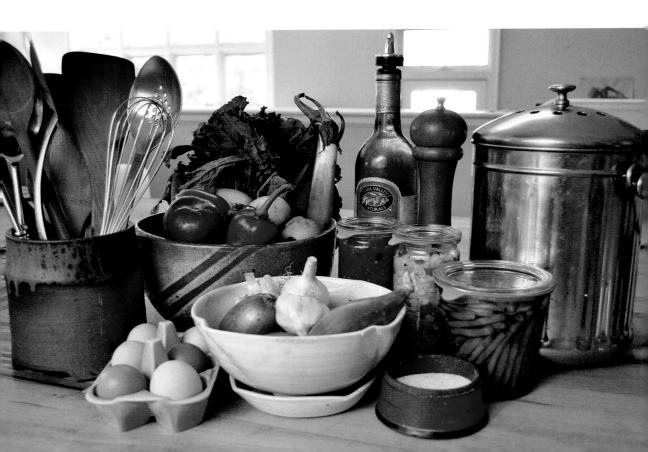

ing you and your children understand all that is required in feeding yourselves. I've heard numerous stories of families who managed to get their kids eating a particular food — carrots or kale for instance — once the kids helped to grow it. These days, almost everyone knows someone raising chickens, hosting bee hives, or sharing a garden patch, and a visit to one of these neighbours can be instructional — even inspirational —to both you and your child.

It is true that you can expect to pay more for quality food, but there is no bargain to be had in getting inferior food at any price savings: real food has a real price. Outside of North America, food is a major household expense. It surpasses the cost of shelter in some countries. Americans spend less of their income on food than people do in most other countries and almost half of that is spent eating out. The habit of unrealistically cheap food spending prioritizes cheap — and often empty — calories over actual nutrients. Think about those university students living on ramen noodles: they can get full on a dollar or two, but they aren't getting nourished. Indeed, when I was in school, there were rumours of kids who developed the severe Vitamin C deficiency, scurvy, from just this habit. While these claims are probably exaggerated, nutritional experts such as Kelly Dorfman say their practices provide numerous examples of middle-class children suffering from malnutrition of one sort or another.

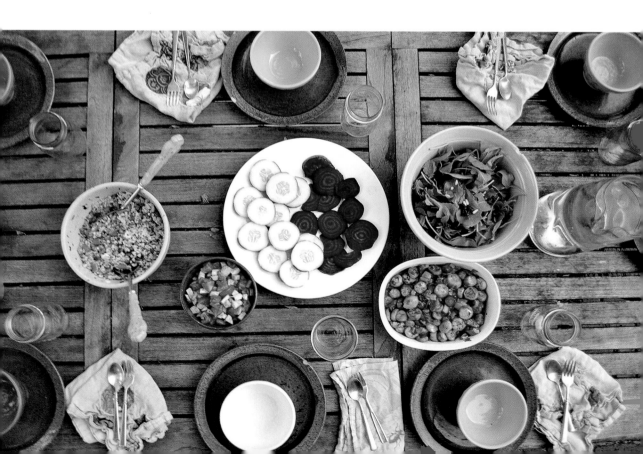

It's also important to cook. Home-cooked meals are likely to be less processed, better quality, and more nutritious. They also cost less than trying to eat "healthy" at a restaurant or using prepackaged foods.

Eating is a social act that can bring families together, so I believe it's important to have family mealtimes. There is research linking eating together as a family with benefits ranging from better performance in school to lower risk of substance abuse and obesity. Start this practice the day you put your child in her highchair for her first meal.

And please don't believe everything you read: The principles of healthy eating have been the same for years. News is only what's new today. Often snippets of health studies are taken out of context and reported as if they are the whole truth. The basis of a healthy diet can seem very confusing because reporters, or corporate interests, announce things like "Margarine lower in deadly saturated fats than butter." And then, thirty years later, "Butter is better: Saturated fats not the killer we thought." Be wary of headlines that seem far afield of what your common sense tells you or are just too good to be true.

Foods that are really healthy for you — the organic apple, pasture-raised cow butter, and kale from your garden — don't have big marketing budgets. If you want real information on healthy food, sit down with a good book, like one of the ones I recommend in the Further Reading section.

The Research

Food research is the subject of numerous hulking volumes, so this little chapter isn't going to cover everything. Instead, it will give you the basics of why eating real foods avoids a lot of risks, the importance of parents learning to read labels to help protect their families from the worst pesticides and food contaminants, and give you enough information to ask good questions.

What happened to food? The dramatic changes since the time of my grandmother's youth can be traced to the industrialization of food production. The earth's population in that time increased from 2.5 billion in 1940 to more than 7 billion today. Gone are the days when a family gets most of their food from their own backyard, or even from their own country. What most people eat now is grown on big factory farms where chickens are kept seven to a cage, pigs never see the light of day, and one crop is grown for hundreds of acres. Pesticides are the new normal. Much of the food production has been pushed overseas, where labour costs less and environmental standards are often minimal. Even the foods we are accustomed to eating have jumped geographical boundaries, as once rare treats like bananas, oranges, and avocados have become North American staples. And today, after packaging and

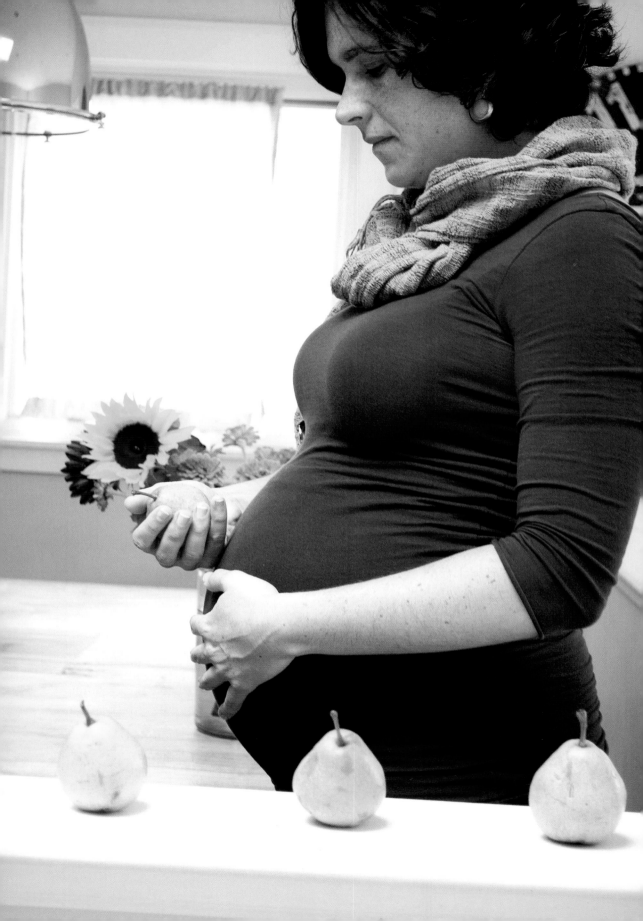

processing, much of what North Americans eat looks nothing like what was grown by the farmer.

We may know that red, waxy, conventional apple is suspicious with its possible residue from one or more of the 42 pesticides used, but our kids are hungry now. Parents are left to do their own research, go the extra distance to the farmers' market, and pay the extra money for the same items grown organically. It is worth it to afford our children the extra protection, but it begs the question: Why isn't it worth it to our governments, elected officials, and corporations to do the same?

The State of Farming Today

Farming is one of the highest petroleum users in the world, one of the biggest polluters, and one of the largest sources of greenhouse gas emissions. Most of these emissions come from farm practices, especially how we raise livestock: all that methane gas that's produced by cows that are eating too much corn instead of grass. For overall pollution, what we eat and how it is raised matters even more than where it comes from.

Since the 1950s, farming has become very dependent on chemicals: 10 of the 12 most dangerous chemicals are pesticides according to the Stockholm Convention on Persistent Organic Pollutants. Yet, every day, the entire population of North America is exposed to pesticides, which include insecticides, herbicides, and fungicides.

These pollutants end up in the soil, the water, and the air. They also end up in our bodies. In *Slow Death by Rubber Duck*, Rick Smith and Bruce Lourie survey the 27 major body-burden studies conducted around the world: 690 people and 500 discreet chemicals. These studies show that everyone is polluted: including newborn babies, who had, on average, 200 industrial chemicals and pollutants in their umbilical cord blood. The good news is that levels of many first-generation organochlorine pesticides that are now banned, like DDT, are finally starting to decrease in younger generations. The bad news is that many other pesticides, such as the popular organophosphate (OP) pesticides that make up 70 percent of current insecticide use, are found at very high levels in almost every person in North America.

Pesticide producers and even our government often dismiss parents' concerns about pesticides, claiming that the amounts used in the United States and Canada are well within safe limits. The "safe" limits for pesticide residue on foods — the maximum residue levels (MRL) —are based on what industry is able to achieve, "not the science of what is healthy," says Eric Darier, ecological farming senior campaigner with Greenpeace International.

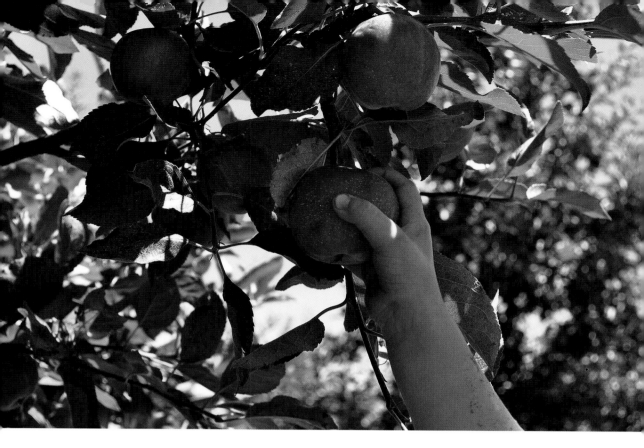

And our children are the most vulnerable — pound for pound they drink two-and-a-half times more water and eat three-to-four times more food — absorbing a higher concentration of pesticides and excreting less than adults. Their developing brains and bodies can be irreversibly damaged by pesticide exposure at the wrong time and pesticides can also block the absorption of important food nutrients necessary for healthy growth.

For instance, take the supposedly safe levels of OP pesticides. A Harvard study found that kids whose typical daily exposure was among the highest were twice as likely to have ADHD. There is research linking pesticide exposure in children to a slew of health effects, including lower IQ, birth defects, neurological disorders, hormonal system disruptions, brain cancer, and leukemia.

The Better, Organic Option

There is some good news, though: parents can help lower their kids' exposure to pesticides and other substances. Children who eat primarily organic produce have one-sixth the levels of pesticide by-products in their urine compared with children who eat conventional produce, according to a study by the University of Washington School of Public Health and Community Medicine.

Organic food may also be more nutritious, according to food scientists at the non-profit research group The Organic Centre, who reviewed more than a hundred studies done on the nutritive value of organic versus conventional food. They concluded that in the majority of cases these plant-based organic foods are more nutritious than their conventional counterparts and can be especially high in some important antioxidants.

Research by the Organic Centre, Consumer Reports, and others suggests that eating organic is an effective strategy for lowering exposure to the pesticides, antibiotics, and artificial growth hormones that can be found in most commercially raised animals.

Problems with Food Additives

There are more than 10,000 chemicals present in food items according to the Pew Charitable Trusts' Food Additives Project. Some are intentionally added to food, while others end up in our food through processing. The FDA and Health Canada are required to assess the safety of food additives before they are used in food, but Pew estimates that only one in five of the chemicals allowed to be directly added to food have ever received even the most basic animal testing; 3,000 of the "approved" chemicals never received any government review; and at least 1,000 of these chemicals are entirely *unknown* to the FDA and the public. Once the FDA and Health Canada have said a food additive or ingredient is "safe," or GRAS, there is little incentive, funding, or demand for adequate research to happen. Many of these too-safe-to-test food additives, including many of those on my list of ones to avoid, don't have to appear anywhere on labels or ingredient lists. Thanks to independent research, we do know some of the more suspicious additives.

The food additives that I suggest you avoid include sugar substitutes such as aspartame and saccharin; artificial food colouring; carrageenan; monosodium glutamate (MSG); partially hydrogenated vegetable oil (trans fat); sodium nitrate/nitrites; and fructose.

Right to Know and Food Labelling

Parents want to know what they are feeding their children. While the world may now be stuck with persistent pesticide residues, GMOs, cloned animals, and lots of artificial food additives, there is growing consumer demand that these items be labelled. "Fifty or 60 countries around the world require labelling of GM foods," says Greenpeace's Eric Darier. This does not include the United States or Canada, however. With labelling, bans become less necessary. "For convenience, retailers won't have one with and one without, so they will go with what consumers want," Darier says. Because of labelling, bans, and import restrictions, when a European consumer — unlike her North American counterpart — reaches for a box of cereal, she will know that it's made without GMO ingredients; when she buys Smarties or M&Ms, it will be clear that they do not contain artificial food colouring; and she'll know that her cheese snacks aren't laced with artificial growth hormone. "If we have a choice, we would rather not eat it," says Darier.

North Americans just want that choice. Whether polled on mandatory labelling of GMOs, artificial growth hormones, irradiation, or cloned animals, it is clear that we want the right to know what is in our food.

"Four years ago, I would have said North America is doomed: nothing will change on food," states Darier. Now, he says he's "moderately optimistic." He points to the upsurge in right-to-know labelling campaigns and the growth in organic agriculture and impassioned local food movements as reasons for hope. Parents can be optimistic too. They are not alone in striving for healthier food for their families. Just remember to think like your great-grandma and don't let packaging, the media, or that nagging thought that "it must be safe because the government wouldn't allow it otherwise," interfere with your common sense.

The ABCs of Food Labels

In North America, at least right now, the only way to know what is in your food is to ensure it contains one of the following labels.

Organic/Biologique

To be able to use the word *organic* on a food label in Canada or the United States, the product must have at least 70 percent organic ingredients and be free of GMOs and the worst of the food additives. A CERTIFIED ORGANIC product contains at least 95 percent organic ingredients, and has an official USDA or CANADA Organic label. These products are grown without chemical herbicides, pesticides, fungicides, fertilizers, sewage sludge, or GMOs. Animals raised organically have access to pasture, eat organic feed containing no antibiotics, and do not receive synthetic growth hormones. The product is not to be irradiated and has no synthetic additives. Canada's organic label has come under criticism recently because, unlike in the United States, Canada does not require field tests and it outsources certifying work that is done in countries such as China that have questionable environmental and business standards. There are additional labels that test the finished food to ensure it is pesticide-free and a label that verifies food is non-GMO.

Green Your Family's Diet

(and Not Go Crazy in the Process)

• •

Here are a series of action steps listed from darkest green (biggest impact, and possibly more work) to lightest green (quick and easy) to get your family eating greener.

- Feed your family like your great grandma did. In my experience it's easier to focus on real foods rather than trying to find packaged or prepared foods that are truly healthy. In my house we eat lentils, a grain, and lots of veggies for at least a thousand meals a week, and breakfast is almost always porridge or eggs. Simple.
- Plant a garden. Even if it's just one pot of herbs, it's amazing to eat something you've grown yourself, and your kids won't grow up believing that food is grown in grocery stores. Even if you don't garden, try to compost. It will cut your garbage almost in half, reduce your greenhouse gas emissions, and you can show your kids where soil comes from.
- Shop your local farmers' market or join a CSA (Community Supported Agriculture) group. CSA boxes come from farms where consumers buy a share of the farm's yield for the season. Typically you pay at the beginning of the growing season for a weekly box of fresh produce delivered to the city. CSAs can be a great bargain, providing farm-fresh, organic produce for about the same price as conventional grocery store produce. And it supports local farmers.
- Buy local, bulk, and direct. When we buy from independent, locally owned businesses, the money we spend translates into double the local economic impact and almost three times the local job creation compared to buying from big box retailers or from restaurant chains. It can also save us money. When buying in bulk or direct from the farmer, the middleman (or three) is cut out, so you and the farmer both benefit.
- Buy organic. When making trade-offs between your budget and organic, prioritize meat, poultry, dairy, eggs, soy, grains, oils, all the fruits and veggies on the Dirty Dozen list (see page 102), and any foods you and your family eat a lot of. The organic label is a handy way to help avoid cloned animal products, irradiation, and GMOs. The organic label also helps to steer us away from products that may contain pesticide residue,

artificial growth hormones, or antibiotics (antibiotic resistance is associated with conventional animal products).

- Know when to look beyond the label. Fish can be great for kids, but you need to ensure that it is low in mercury (not canned tuna) and antibiotics (not farmed salmon) and that it is harvested or raised ecologically. *Kidsafeseafood.org* gives the best ratings to anchovies, farmed arctic char, farmed oysters, farmed rainbow trout, wild Alaskan salmon (chum, coho, and sockeye), wild Atlantic mackerel, and wild sardines. As well, be wary of processed meats, such as hotdogs, salami, and lunch meats, even if they are labelled "natural." High levels of nitrates can still be found in meat products claiming to have "all natural ingredients" and "no added preservatives." There is research linking processed meat consumption to pancreatic cancer, brain tumours in children (even when eaten by mom during pregnancy), and a 700 percent increase in the chance of developing leukemia.

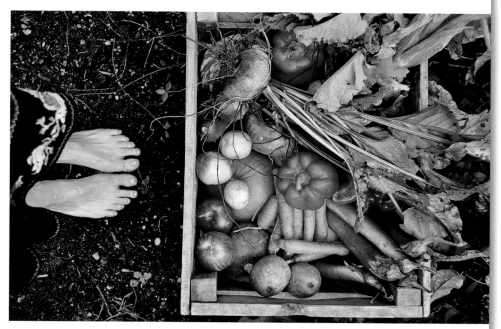

- Serve good-quality fats. Brains are composed of 60 percent fat, more than a third of which is the essential fatty acid DHA. If the brain doesn't have enough of this high quality fat, it will substitute a lesser quality fat. Essential fatty acids are fats that the body can't make on its own and must be consumed. EFAs are found in fish, fish oil, seaweed, olive oil, seeds, and nuts. Two of the most important EFAs are omega-3 and omega-6. Most people have an excess of omega-6s (which can come from vegetable oils) and don't have enough omega-3s. This imbalance can cause inflammation in the body and lead to heart disease and other issues. The best oils for all people, especially children, include animal fats, coconut oil, butter, olive oil, and oils containing omega-3s (such as cod liver or krill oil). Remember fats should always be from the highest quality source possible: organic and free-range. Avoid margarines, palm oil, canola oil, corn oil, and other vegetable and seed oils, which may lead to inflammation, arterial damage, and are inadequate for the important work of brain development.

- Filter your water. An average glass of tap water can contain residue from 44 or more pesticides. A lot of tap water also contains lead from old pipes. The CBC reported that "even sophisticated water treatment systems are helpless when it comes to removing pesticides, pharmaceuticals, antibiotics and hormones." But please don't take this information and go running to the open arms of the bottled water industry. Bottled water has fewer regulations protecting it than tap water, and, in addition, it devastates the environment, using 1.5 million barrels of oil a year. Plasticizers can leach from some bottles, further polluting the water. Buying bottled water would cost a family of four over $1,200 year. Instead, invest in a good water filtration system for your home and carry either a glass or stainless steel bottle for drinking.

- Invest in your kitchen. It will be easier to cook for yourself if you have a few good-quality essentials. These include: a slow-cooker (ceramic, not non-stick, interior); cast iron, stainless steel, ceramic-coated, or titanium pots and pans; stainless steel and wooden kitchen utensils; storage containers made from glass and or stainless steel; and a small, energy-efficient deep freezer so you can stockpile your abundance. Avoid all non-stick cookware, it uses the "likely carcinogenic" PFC (new "green" non-stick cookware options simply uses a less-tested, but structurally similar chemical).

- Learn a few cooking and food saving tricks. For instance, you can freeze all sorts of foods. Make a huge pot of chili and then freeze half of it. It's not much more work and it's twice the meals. You can use this trick to take advantage of sales and seasonal favourites. You can even freeze dairy products. Learn to make your own stock: bone broth in particular is a great source of calcium and other minerals and you can make it from the parts that are usually considered "left-over." You can make a vegetarian version from vegetable scraps, too. It's much healthier than the prepared concentrate, powder, or cubes. Try freezing your broth in stainless steel ice-cube trays to make a healthy alternative to a bouillon cube. You can throw all of this in your freezer along with other essentials like containers of pre-soaked beans, sticks of butter, and waffles you made yourself.

- Pack your kids' lunches. This is particularly important in the United States, where the USDA sources food for the national school lunch program with items that consumers wouldn't otherwise buy. They also consider french fries, the tomato paste on pizza, and pickle relish to meet the required vegetable servings. See if you can make her lunch waste-free with reusable sandwich bags, a stainless steel thermos, and a cloth napkin.

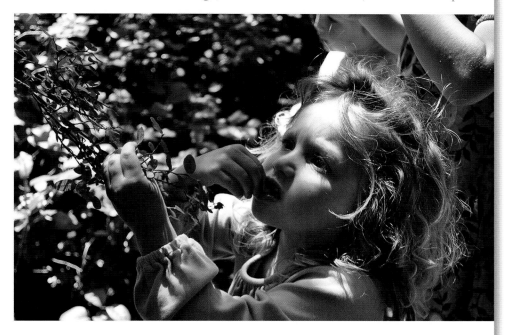

- Don't keep junk food around. If you don't have crackers in your cupboard, you won't feed them to your children. The same goes for all processed foods. Skip the interior of the grocery store where most of the packaged food is sold. This strategy has turned me into a person who reaches for the fresh apple instead of the bag of chips.
- Don't routinely drink juice, soda, or sports drinks. Drinks, even the kinds without added sugar, are basically empty calories and usually loaded with fructose. Fructose triggers the body to make fat and blocks its ability to burn fat. It also depletes energy and triggers hunger. Most people today eat or drink about 600 more sugar calories daily than when I was young: an average child consumes 34 teaspoons of sugar every day. The more we eat — or drink — the more our bodies crave, says researcher Dr. Robert Ludwig, author of *Fat Chance*. He suggests

this addictive behaviour can start before kids are even born, crossing the placenta and programming the unborn baby to crave sugar. He specifically warns against infant formula, juices, and sweetened milks, all of which can make kids fat. Even no-sugar-added juice can contain as much sugar as a cola, he says. Juice is not the same as eating fresh fruit. Not only do you drink more of the sugar because it is concentrated, but you also take the fibre away, which slows the absorption.

- Eat out less. Eating out just once less a week can save the average American one eighth of their food budget. It is also harder to eat out well. Restaurant food is less likely to be organic, more like to contain GMOs, and it's harder to avoid the food additives. Meals from restaurants and fast food sources also tend to be less nutritious because they rely less on fresh fruits and vegetables.

- Avoid food in packages. Packaging increases chemical exposure in what might otherwise be healthy food: this includes food and drinks that come in cans or plastic and restaurant takeout that has been placed into Styrofoam or plastic containers or wrapped in non-stick paper. Foods eaten from Styrofoam or melamine plates or microwaved in plastic or non-stick wrappers can be contaminated by their packaging. There is evidence to suggest that even your potato chip bag, candy wrapper, and that paper cup for hot beverages can leach toxins.

- Follow your intuition. Our grandmothers had less education, but they fed their children healthy foods. Cut through the confusion by channelling grandma and by getting educated. According to Kelly Dorfman, author of *How to Cure Your Child with Food*, "The key is to get clear. I never fought with my kids about this because for me it was clear and thus they were comfortable. We fought about stuff that I wasn't sure about, like when do you get your ears pierced."

Cage-Free, Free-Range, Grass-Fed, Hormone-Free, Antibiotic-Free, Natural or All-Natural

If I see one of these terms being used without a certifying body backing it up or without knowing the farmer, I assume the company is greenwashing, as the government does not provide oversight on these terms. For meat from animals that have been given access to grass pastureland and allowed free range, look for the Animal Welfare Approved (AWA) label. For eggs from hens that get to spend time running around outdoors, rather than locked inside overcrowded barns and fed antibiotics, look for eggs labelled AWA, or certified by the Canadian Organic Regime, the Certified Organic Association of BC, Pro-Cert, or BC SPCA (with the exception of those labelled "Free-Run," which means they are given area to run around only indoors). For truly antibiotic-free animal products there must be a "USDA Process Verified" label along with the "No Antibiotics Administered" label or a USDA/CANADA Organic label, which also guarantees the meat is hormone-free. *Natural* does not mean an animal wasn't fed antibiotics or hormones, nor does it mean the food wasn't processed with nitrates or other food additives.

Fair Trade

FLO-CERT and Fair to Life are two organizations that certify products, or ingredients, to ensure that farmers, mostly in the developing world, are paid a living wage and are treated fairly. They support co-operatives and family farms and minimize middlemen. Their growers use sustainable farming practices with limited agrochemicals and no GMOs.

Sustainable Seafood

The USDA and CANADA Organic labels are currently meaningless when it comes to fish, so be wary when you see seafood labelled as organic. Proposed standards are on the way. In the meantime, other labels exist to indicate you are getting fish that was caught with respect to the health of the oceans, was not cloned or fed GMO food, and wasn't treated with the heavy doses of antibiotics fed to most farm-raised fish. Unfortunately, none of the current labels for seafood are very rigorous. The Marine Stewardship Council label indicates that seafood is wild-caught and the fishery is practising a minimum of care. The Monterey Bay Aquarium has Seafood Watch, which provides guides, by region, and Canadians have a similar system called SeaChoice. Canadians also have the Vancouver Aquarium's Ocean Wise certification found at many West Coast restaurants. Greenpeace posts a Redlist of the most endangered fish species on its website. All of these labels focus on the environment, however. To find seafood that is lower in mercury and other contaminants, Seafood Watch maintains a Super Green List and the KidSafeSeafood program reports seafood choices that are gentler on both Earth and body.

— green tip —

Secrets of a Produce Detective

You can "decode" the PLU code to decipher the food in your grocery store. If the code begins with 9 it's organic, 4 it's conventional, 8 it's genetically engineered.

"The Dirty Dozen"

The dirty dozen refers to the fruits and vegetables that have the highest levels of pesticide residue. My favourite resource is the EWG because they look at both the most contaminated produce and the cleaner alternatives. The foods in their samples are washed before being tested. Don't assume washing or peeling a food improves its ranking: many pesticides are absorbed by the plants as is the water and nutrients from the soil.

And the Dirty Dozen are:

1. Peaches/nectarines/apples/pears/plums (and other orchard fruits)
2. Celery
3. Berries, including strawberries, blueberries, cherries, and red raspberries
4. Tomatoes
5. Sweet bell peppers and hot peppers
6. Leafy greens, including spinach, kale, collard greens, and lettuce
7. Potatoes
8. Grapes (especially imported)
9. Carrots
10. Summer squash, zucchini
11. Cucumbers
12. Hawaiian pineapples

The fruits and vegetables that are generally less contaminated include onions, avocado, asparagus, frozen sweet peas, mango, kiwi, domestic cantaloupe, and sweet potatoes.

Becoming a Nutrition Detective

Kelly Dorfman is a nutrition detective and author of *How to Cure Your Child with Food*. She works with hard to crack cases: parents who have already taken their children to see numerous doctors to try to determine what's behind symptoms such as rashes, chronic colds, sleep problems, and developmental delays. She stresses that parents may suspect a diet-related issue, but are often talked out of trusting their instincts.

Foods can become problems in two ways, says Dorfman: "Either something is missing from the diet or something in the diet is aggravating the body. The first step is to get your child eating real food," says Dorfman. This means whole foods, lots of fresh fruits and vegetables, and maybe some additional supplemental sources for essential fatty acids and vitamins. "Crackers are like toddler

crack," she warns. Crackers and cookies fill kids up but don't give them what
they need to thrive. Remember: "Picky eating isn't normal."

The second step to becoming a food detective is elimination. The first things
to try eliminating from a diet include any foods parents suspect are problematic,
junk foods, and the major allergens: dairy, sugar, gluten, wheat, soy, and corn.
Eliminate the possible irritant for four to six weeks. Keep a log. If the child gets
only a bit better, try eliminating the next thing on the list as well.

Got Milk?

Most people are told their entire lives that milk is healthy and that low-fat milk
is healthiest. Certainly, kids need it to develop healthy bones and all that, right?
Even Health Canada and the USDA recommend that children (and adults) drink
two to three glasses of reduced-fat milk every day. Yet, these recommendations
are not borne out by research. There is no nutritional requirement for animal
milk, other than human breast milk. We're told that milk is necessary to "build

strong bones," yet the higher the milk consumption in a country, the higher the bone fracture rates. And reduced-fat milk not only fails to guard against weight gain, some studies associate it with equal or greater weight gain. It may also raise cholesterol more than whole milk.

Even more troubling is the connection between the intake of low-fat dairy foods and an increase in infertility. A study led by Dr Jorge Chavarro from the Harvard School of Public Health examined 18,555 married, premenopausal women between the ages of 24 and 42 with no history of infertility and found a connection between low-fat dairy consumption and infertility.

Looking at the evidence, I strongly recommend that parents feed their children unprocessed, organic, full-fat dairy. Chocolate milk, especially reduced-fat varieties, is a bad idea. Women trying to get pregnant should avoid all low-fat dairy products. Isn't it amazing when science recommends what your tongue always told you? The yummier stuff is actually better for you.

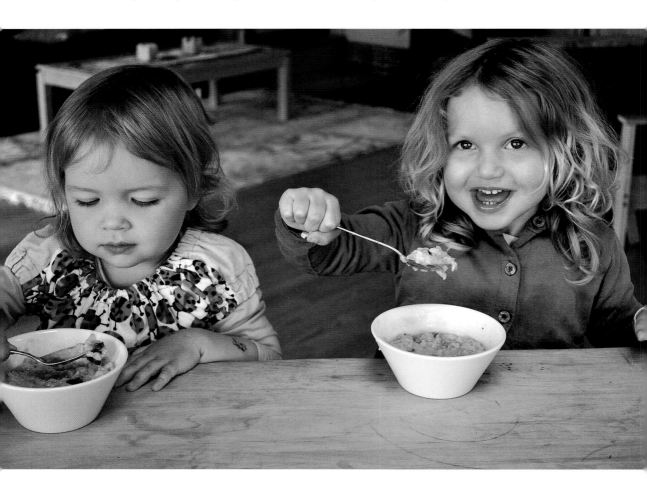

chapter five

Greening Skincare

• •

It was a gift: an expensive, foaming pump bottle of "Gentle! For Bebe!" shampoo. It was French, so I thought it wouldn't contain carcinogens, neurotoxins, or allergens. I used it on my baby for two years before I thought to take a closer look at the ingredients. When I finally squinted hard at that super-tiny ingredient list (*is that written in English?*) I knew it was bad, even without referencing my "cheat sheet": synthetic fragrances, four different parabens, phenoxyethanol, and a number of other frightening-sounding ingredients.

Start counting now. How many personal care (or beauty) products have you used already today? Cleanser for your face, toothpaste, shampoo, conditioner, shaving cream, deodorant, lotion, mascara, lipstick, makeup remover, something for that blemish.... What about your child? Diaper cream, baby wipes, sunscreen, soap, baby powder …

Cosmetic ingredients do not stay on the surface of the skin — they are designed to penetrate, and they do. What we put on our skin can be absorbed and go directly into our bloodstream. So if it's been days since you showered or used deodorant, you might be luckier than you realize, as most products in your medicine cabinet contain at least one potentially toxic ingredient. The average woman applies more than five hundred chemicals daily, and many of these are known or suspected carcinogens, neurotoxins, hormone mimickers, allergens, and environmental toxins. And she will spend upward of a thousand dollars a year for the pleasure.

But children's products are safer, right? In fact, 77 percent of the ingredients in 17,000 reviewed children's products have never been assessed for safety by industry or government. The average baby is exposed daily to 27 untested chemicals in his baby care products alone. Diaper wipes can contain parabens, perfumes, and numerous unintended contaminants, like the known human carcinogen formaldehyde and the possibly carcinogenic 1,4-dioxane. A study done by the Campaign for Safer Cosmetics (CSC) looked at 28 common beauty products sold for children

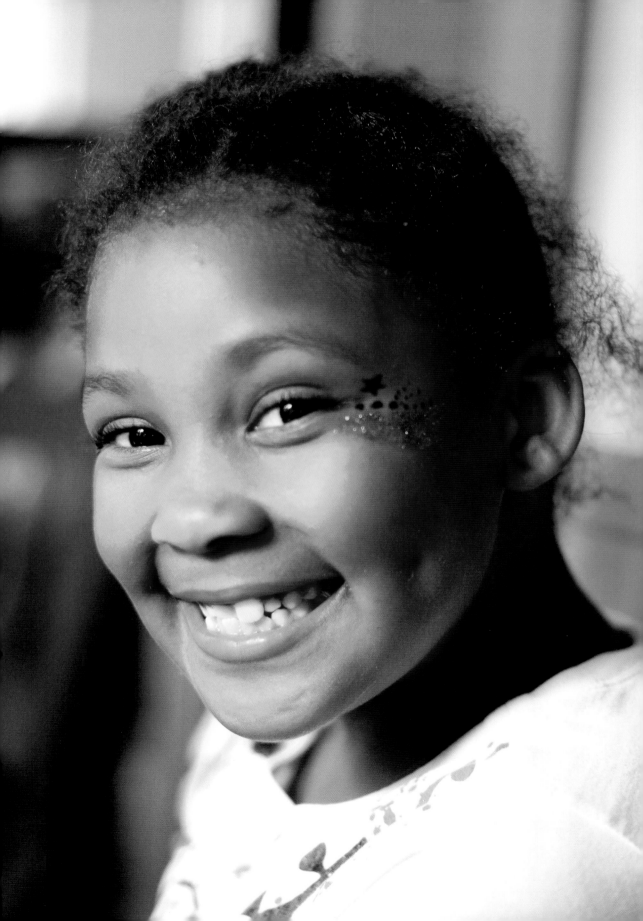

and found that 82 percent contained traces of formaldehyde and more than half contained both formaldehyde and 1,4-dioxane. What's a parent to do?

Think Like an Earth Mama Beauty Queen

Fortunately, the mindset of a green beauty queen is quite simple: use food. Basic ingredients should be so pure that they are food-grade and so few that you can count them on one hand. If a label is full of lots of unpronounceable ingredients, don't assume they were put in there by experts who know what your baby needs. Assume that the product isn't good enough for your baby.

If you still want that product, apply the sniff test. If it smells like perfume or makes you sneeze, take a pass. Synthetic fragrance can contain some of the worst neurotoxins, allergens, and even phthalates (and stating on the label that something is "unscented" doesn't mean perfume hasn't been added). Perfumes are a clue that a product isn't as natural, green, healthy, or baby-safe as you expect it to be.

And remember: Less is more. Babies have extremely porous skin and they don't detoxify. So be super careful about what goes in those pores. All that is necessary is gentle soap and water to clean the diaper area when you change or potty your child, an occasional warm bath, and, when they need a little extra protection from the elements or their diaper, try pure virgin olive oil, coconut oil, or cocoa butter. (Yummy!)

Beware of "greenwashing": it's everywhere in the beauty care industry. Don't be fooled (like I was) by European brands or safe-sounding words or phrases such as *non-toxic*, *safe*, *hypo-allergenic*, *for baby*, or *organic* (unless it is USDA certified). These words aren't regulated and are thus meaningless. Look for products with the USDA Organic seal or those from small companies with whom you can talk to ensure the freshness and health of the item.

Or best of all, make your own beauty products. This can be as simple as rubbing oil on your baby as mentioned above or using the DIY recipes in this chapter for bum balms, lotions, and even sunscreen.

The Research

It's a fact: Most of what we put *on* our bodies ends up *in* our bodies. Every body-burden study ever done has found that many of the ingredients in personal care products bioaccumulate inside our bodies and end up in our bloodstreams. Babies are born with dozens of these ingredients already in them, inherited from their mothers.

The amount and speed of absorption of these substances depend largely on their molecular weight. Many synthetic preservatives and fragrances added to skincare products are designed to be readily absorbed through the skin, while whole, food-grade oils have a high molecular weight and tend to stay on the surface where they can moisturize the skin.

In addition to breathing more and not having the ability to fully detoxify, children have skin that is thinner and absorbs more of what it contacts than adults do. The EPA calculates that carcinogens are typically ten times more potent for babies and some chemicals up to 65 times more potent for children. And, as parents know, children put arms, feet, hands (dirty or "clean"), and pretty much anything they can get their hands on, into their mouths.

Chemicals over Generations

Our mothers and grandmothers didn't use as many products on themselves or their children as most of us do today, nor did those products contain as many potentially harmful ingredients. The United States alone approves an average of seven new chemicals every day and has more than 85,000 chemicals in commerce, according to the California Department of Toxic Substance Control. We've gotten really good at creating effective new substances that can do amazing things — *Look! It's non-stick! It's flexible and strong! It holds smell forever!*

Some of these new substances can also do amazingly bad things, such as disrupt normal hormone function (endocrine disruptors). Even more alarming, some have transgenerational effects: when animals are exposed in utero, the effects are transmitted not only to the immediate offspring, but are inherited by future generations.

Though limited, there are some human studies. Women exposed to the anti-miscarriage drug diethylstilbestrol (DES) passed down an increased risk of a variety of abnormalities and diseases, from hip dysplasia to irregular periods, to their granddaughters. Women exposed to famine-like food restrictions during pregnancy had grandchildren at higher risk for certain neurological, autoimmune, and dermatological conditions. The study of transgenerational effects — epigenetics — is relatively new, and it is not fully understood *how* these effects are passed down through the generations. It is neither easy nor fast to study the effects of chemicals on humans over generations, but there have been transgenerational effects based on animal studies reported for a variety of chemicals already, including BPA, certain phthalates, dioxin, and many more.

Beauty Care Is Big Business

Beauty care is big business, with $170 billion spent annually on skincare, hair care, perfume, sunscreen, makeup, toothpaste, deodorant, and other personal care items.

The global demand for "organic" personal care products is expected to reach US$13.2 billion by 2018. As consumers begin to demand healthier personal care products, many of the big players are trying to capitalize. They own brands that seem smaller and more natural: Clorox owns Burt's Bees; Colgate-Palmolive owns Tom's of Maine; L'Oréal owns The Body Shop; and Estée Lauder owns Aveda.

Unfortunately, lack of government oversight makes it hard to determine which personal care brands are truly green and which are just faking it. Consumers have a growing interest in healthier baby products especially, and are willing to pay more for products that are truly pure. Sales of premium/organic baby care items are fast-growing, with a 68 percent increase in America from 2005 to 2010, according to the market-research company Euromonitor International, which also forecasts sales continuing to grow through 2017.

Unfortunately, many companies have been caught using the same old dangerous formulas but advertising them as more natural and selling them, naturally,

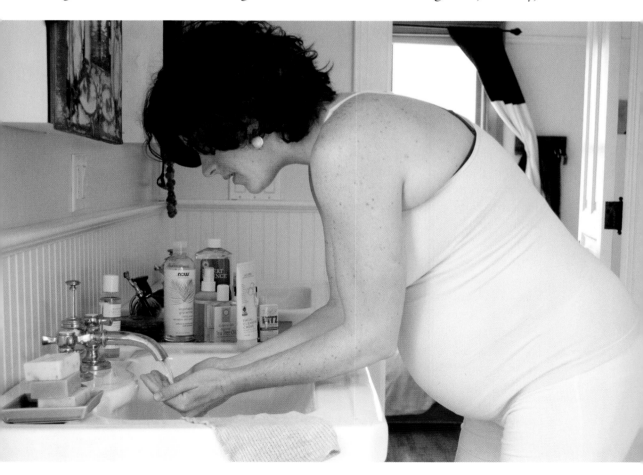

for a higher price. Non-governmental organizations such as the CSC, Greenpeace, and Organic Consumers Association have made headway getting some of these corporations to start cleaning up their acts: Johnson & Johnson committed to reformulating its baby products to remove 1,4-dioxane and formaldehyde releasers, and Target, in collaboration with the CSC, has agreed to start ranking ingredient safety on products in their personal care aisle. Whole Foods has led the way in cleaning up the beauty care aisle by forcing the brands they carry to certify their organic claims. Uncertified claims, including when it appears as part of a beauty product's name, aren't allowed.

Government Oversight Is Lacking

The move toward more natural alternatives in personal care comes in the wake of non-governmental organizations' research and reports on the dangerous chemicals allowed in current products. As consumers, and especially women, began to hear about the relatively high levels of known toxins in their cosmetics, such as lead in lipstick and mercury in mascara, it became clear that we were on our own.

There may be change afoot. In Canada, cosmetics are required to list their ingredients on the label; however, there is a major loophole. Regulations don't require the full disclosure of ingredients for anything considered to have a therapeutic purpose, including antiperspirants, hand sanitizers, and toothpaste. Nor does Canada require labelling on the hundreds of ingredients in fragrances/perfumes.

Health Canada does maintain a Hotlist of restricted and prohibited ingredients, but this list is not enforced because it has no legal authority. The list also excludes unintentional ingredients or impurities. For instance, while formaldehyde is a known human carcinogen that appears on the Hotlist, there are a number of commonly used cosmetic preservatives, such as DMDM hydantoin, that release formaldehyde, but they do not appear on the list.

While the United States still does not require labelling of cosmetic ingredients, they do have California's Proposition 65, the Safe Drinking Water and Toxic Enforcement Act of 1986, which requires the government to publish a list of chemicals known to be carcinogens and/or reproductive toxicants. Any cosmetic product sold in the state that contains an ingredient on the list must be reported and properly labelled. Prop 65 is enforceable by the state and has already resulted in a number of significant lawsuits and fines.

The EU goes further with REACH, the "Registration, Evaluation, Authorization and restriction of Chemicals." The law requires manufacturers and importers of chemicals to both identify and manage risks linked to these substances and to promote the use of safer alternatives to hazardous substances. REACH goes beyond labelling to allow the government to restrict

"There's Lead in My Lipstick"

Gill Deacon is the author of my favourite book on green beauty: *There's Lead in Your Lipstick*. It's full of great information and tips. (Did you know it's possible to get rid of cellulite with used coffee grounds?!) She is also a TV broadcaster and the host of *Here and Now* on CBC radio. She speaks with the wisdom of having three young boys and having survived cancer. She knows what it's like trying to walk the green tightrope. Despite all her work in this field, her eldest son came home this summer with a chemical-laden, super stinky, toxic deodorant. She laughed: "He knows that I am allergic to it, he knows it is full of super icky chemicals, but he is at the stage of his life where he is testing boundaries." At home he still uses the other green body care products she has provided around the house, but in this area he gave in to peer pressure. She cautions moms to "not become hysterical about it." But she knows that's hard: "There is so much awareness … what's lurking at every corner, in every toy … you can become a little paranoid.

"The idea of creating a perfect world for our babies is so appealing. It's natural for a mother to try and carve out an environment that is pure for her offspring. That's biology at work. Yet, it's incredibly taxing on the mother, stressful for the household, and kids pick up on that stress," Gill says. She encourages all people to inform themselves about ingredients and find the real ones whenever possible. She also says it's about "maintaining that perspective: we are never going to have everything perfect or everything in control: you can have the most perfect, organic household and your kid can still walk out the door in the morning and inhale benzene from the cars driving by. The stress of trying to keep everything perfect will probably kill you first."

the manufacture and marketing of substances found to pose an unacceptable risk to human health or the environment. These more effective regulatory systems provide a model of what is possible and prove that consumers can spur changes in what may seem like a huge industry.

Organic Beauty Care Labels Demystified

With so little oversight of beauty care, many parents are looking for certifying bodies that will tell them what is really safe. But labels have virtually no meaning when it comes to body care products. These labels may include: "natural," "non-toxic," "hypoallergenic," "doctor recommended," "safe for baby," "herbal," or even (wait for it....) "organic." I know, I know. Didn't I just say in the food section that if a product uses organic, it must be verified and contain 95 percent organic ingredients? Yes, but that only applies to *food ingredients*.

A cosmetic product, like that leaded lipstick or that formalehyde-containing baby shampoo, might have every single one of those green-sounding soothing words on its label. It's allowed in North America because body care product labels aren't regulated by either the USDA or Health Canada, the agencies that oversee food labels. If a beauty care product is made from all organic food ingredients, it could receive the USDA organic label, but the Canadian "organic/biologique" label is not supposed to be applied to body care products.

Skincare Labels You Can Trust

What do you do when you're standing in the aisle desperately trying to read the fine print while your child is pulling at your leg and your baby is screaming in the buggy? Thankfully, there are short-cut labels and USDA Organic is considered the North American gold-standard for safer cosmetics. In order for a product to get the USDA Organic seal, it must contain at least 95 percent organic food-grade ingredients and the other non-organic ingredients are restricted to safer options. European or internationally recognized labels of a similar high-quality standard include BDIH, the NaTrue three-star rating, and ACO and NASAA in Australia.

If you are just concerned that the tea tree oil in that shampoo is really organic, there are a number of third-party labels that are used to certify the "made with organic ingredients" claim but allow a number of synthetics and more processing (thus more impurities). These certifying bodies include the NSF in the United States. In the EU, several major labels — including EcoCert and the Soil Association — came together to create COSMOS (COSMetic Organic Standard).

— green tip —

More Products to Avoid

Fluoride should be avoided until children can reliably not swallow the toothpaste. Sunscreen should be avoided for babies younger than six months old. And talcum or baby powder should not be used on children as it can harm their developing lungs if inhaled.

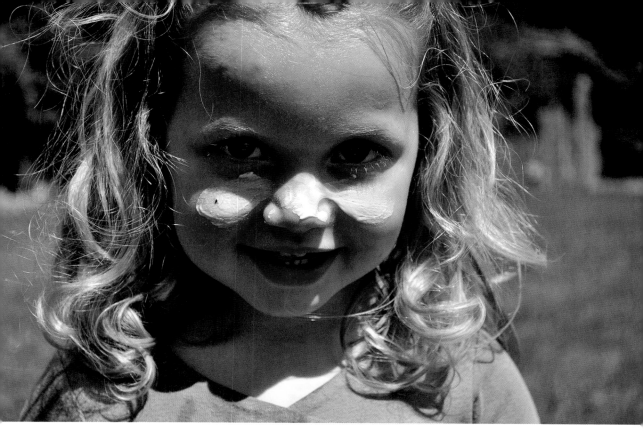

And Then There's Sunscreen ...

Sunscreen will really put your label-reading skills to the test. The most important tip is to "eat your sunscreen": foods high in sun-protective carotenoid phytonutrients such as dark, leafy greens, yellow-orange fruits, and vegetables like carrots and apricots. Other good sources include eggs, spirulina, and wild salmon. Vitamin D can help prevent cellular damage from the sun. It comes from daily moderate sun exposure and from animals that have themselves been exposed to sunlight or, in the case of fatty fishes, have eaten phytoplankton.

For the stuff you slather on your baby, the most effective sunscreens rely on mineral ingredients, like zinc oxide, that aren't foods. So they won't get the USDA Organic label that you look for on most of your other cosmetics.

Sunscreen is not as straightforward as our mothers once thought. This is because the evidence suggests that sunscreen alone is not that effective at protecting us from deadliest skin cancer: malignant melanoma. In 2007, the FDA hinted at these troubles when it said it was "not aware of data demonstrating that sunscreen use alone helps prevent skin cancer." In the same year, a review of literature led by award-winning cancer researcher Dr. Ed Gorham was published in the *Annals of Epidemiology*. It reviewed 17 (out of 18 known) studies on the subject and concluded that "there was no statistically significant effect of use of sunscreens on risk of melanoma." He also theorized that the use of "common sunscreen formulations" may "contribute to risk of melanoma in populations at latitudes >40 degrees."

How is it possible for sunscreen use to increase skin cancer risk for us poor northerners? One theory, proposed by Dr. Gorham's team, is that, because sunscreens aren't so good at blocking UVA rays but are quite effective at blocking UVB rays, the skin doesn't noticeably burn, but it still gets zapped with the UVA. Another theory is that some sunscreen users may develop a false sense of security and end up staying in the sun longer, especially when using products with a high SPF rating. Studies suggest that this may increase their skin cancer risk.

Broad-spectrum sunscreens are now being designed to protect against both types of rays, but most still aren't as effective at protecting against UVA.

These problems with sunscreen don't even take into account that many sunscreens contain known cancer-causing ingredients. Independent researchers at the EWG reviewed 500 popular sunscreens and recommended only 39 of them as safe for consumers. The worst offenders were often the market leaders, and none received a perfect score. Many brands made inaccurate and misleading claims such as "waterproof," "broad-spectrum protection," and even "chemical-free." Other claims to be wary of include "for babies," "natural," and any SPF over 50.

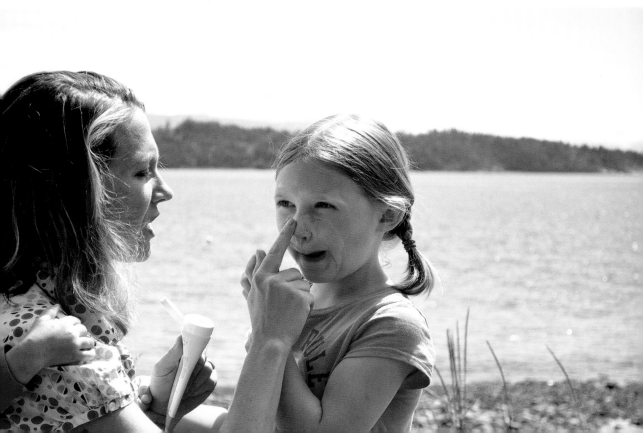

In the United States and Canada, sunscreens are regulated as drugs. This means that products making sunscreen claims are not required to list all of their ingredients on the labels in either country. It also means it has taken longer for both countries to approve some of the newer ingredients currently in use in the EU and Japan that may be safer and provide more UVA protection.

There are two types of sunscreen readily available. Chemical sunscreens rely on chemicals to filter UV rays. The most commonly used of these filters, oxybenzone, can cause allergic skin reactions and may disrupt hormones. Mineral sunscreens are also available. They generally rely on zinc oxide and titanium dioxide to block UV rays. Mineral sunscreens are considered safer, but the ones proven safest — and best at blocking the UVA rays — tend to leave you with that thick white sheen you may remember from the lifeguards of your childhood. In order to get away from that look, many sunscreens use these minerals in nanoparticle form. But this means the ingredients are so small that there is the possibility that they may enter the bloodstream. Research on their safety is currently lacking. Studies have shown that nano-titanium dioxide found in some sunscreens is destroying important microbes found in aquatic ecosystems and that they may be toxic to aquatic life.

What I suggest you look for in sunscreen:

- Mineral sunscreens: the bigger the particle size, the better, but companies aren't required to reveal this information in North America.
- Sunscreens that provide "broad spectrum" protection.

What to avoid:

- Any of the following ingredients: oxybenzone, PABA, or retinyl palmitate (which was found to speed up the development of cancerous lesions and tumours on UV-treated animals in a study conducted by the NTP).
- SPFs higher than 50; the FDA warns that this can mean the product is loaded with more of the most hazardous ingredients and doesn't actually provide any more protection. It's better to use an SPF between 15 and 50 and reapply frequently and generously.
- Spray sunscreens. When sunscreen is sprayed, it can be inhaled, where it can do damage to the lungs. Even mineral sunscreens aren't safe in spray form, as titanium dioxide becomes a "possible carcinogen" when inhaled in high doses.

Greenwashing: How Little White Lies Can Harm

Greenwashing exploits the language of "green" to make a product or company appear healthier for people and the planet than it really is. For example, you walk into the grocery aisle to find a baby shampoo that contains no unwanted, potentially toxic ingredients. You look at bottles labelled "Hypoallergenic," "No Tears," "Dermatologist-tested," "Natural," "Organic," and even "Safe for Baby." Lucky you, there it is: a bottle with ALL of these on the label. It's two dollars more than the one next to it, but it's worth it, right?

What happens then when you get home and actually have two minutes to read the ingredients? There you discover your expensive, green-sounding product is loaded with those very ingredients you were trying to avoid.

They lied, you think.

No, they greenwashed. They misled you into thinking their product was green, they charged you more, and yet they gave you the same old formula. Greenwashing is BIG business, with lots of consumer dollars to be won: "green" accounts for some of the fastest-growing sectors in food, building, and personal care products. The researchers at The Sins of Greenwashing say that 95 percent of companies are doing some greenwashing. Yikes. It really helps when consumers stop buying products from companies that greenwash and switch over to the companies really doing a better job.

Perhaps the saddest cases are those in which formerly great companies go bad: it may be accidental, or it may happen when they change ownership, or they get

When Money Matters More

Trying to buy greener personal care products with little money can be frustrating, especially in a remote community where there simply is nowhere to buy better commercial products. I've been going with my young children to Guatemala for the last three years and every single place only sells antibacterial pump soap, fragrance-laden shampoos, and lotions that seem to have extra carcinogens added just to drive me crazy.

There is a silver lining when it comes to personal care products: less is truly more. Children need virtually nothing added to their skin to stay clean, healthy, and vibrant: a little pure soap, an occasional balm for their bums, a bit of shampoo every so often. If finding healthier options is difficult, go to the grocery aisle of your local store. Just about any grocery store now will stock good oils and maybe a basic castile soap.

so big that profits become more important than social responsibility. It's why you can never give up the habit of reading labels, and why I am always reluctant to "name names." Brands that I have loved in the past, but stopped using when I found out that some less-than-green ingredients had made their way into their products, include Aveda, Burt's Bees, The Body Shop, and Method. The Organic Consumer Association and Consumers Union filed a legal petition in 2010 requesting action on the blatantly deceptive labelling or advertising practices of several "organic" personal care brands.

Funky Fingernails

Many kids love to paint their nails and parents may also use nail polish or nail-biting deterrents to discourage nail-biting or thumb-sucking. Nail polish can be full of some of the worst toxins on the list. There are safer water-based, pealable alternatives available, although these can still contain artificial dyes and/or glycol ethers. You can rub a little virgin olive oil on the nail to help lessen the amount absorbed into the body. All the commercial available nail-biting deterrents contain numerous harmful ingredients and should be avoided.

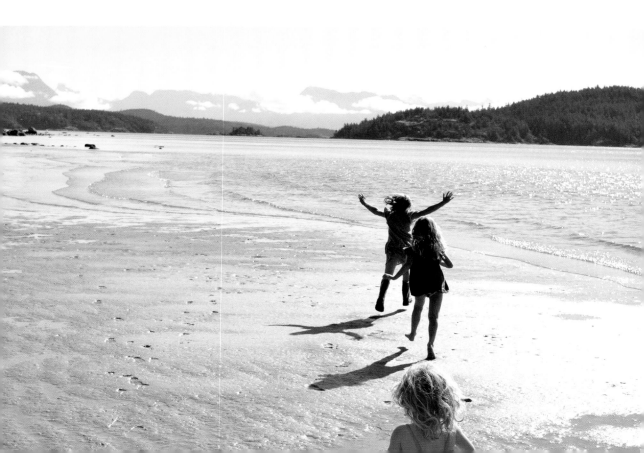

Green Your Child's Skincare

(and Make It Edible!)

• •

Here are a series of action steps listed from darkest green (biggest impact, possibly more work) to lightest green (quick and easy) to making sure your child's kept healthy from the outside in.

- Choose baby skincare carefully. View with suspicion products you can't eat or your great grandma didn't use. Use the simplest food-grade products you can find on your baby (including food itself, like organic oils) and stay open to the possibility that you need them less often than marketing leads us to believe.

- DIY for complete quality control. You can make everything you need yourself: lotions, shampoos, sunscreen, deodorant, and more. It's easy and fun, like cooking from a simple recipe, and it is especially rewarding as a project shared with other parents. There are likely some moms making really pure, food-grade cosmetics in a kitchen near you, or check out your local farmer's market, co-op, or look on *www.etsy.com*.

- Read labels. This is an essential skill of green parenting, especially for all personal care items. I have gotten really good at remembering just three items on the long list of scary chemical additives: fragrances, anything with paraben, and anything that claims to be antibacterial (see Appendix 2 for the complete list). There's a good chance that if these are present, other yucky ingredients are in there too. Treat greenwashing with disdain. Claims like: "Natural!" "Made with real lavender!" "Doctor recommended!" make me laugh when I read them. If it's not backed by the USDA Organic label, it might be a sign the company is trying to fake it.

- Practise safe sun protection. Get good sun clothing for your child: a sunhat, a full-body bathing suit, and long-sleeved light shirts. When you buy sunscreen, something bad isn't better than nothing. Unfortunately, the safest sunscreens for your child are often white and goopy. Young kids typically don't mind though. For me, I usually get something tinted to wear along with my sunhat so that it is more like makeup.

- Avoid ALL antibacterial soaps and sanitizers. If your child's daycare provider, preschool, or other school is using antibacterial hand soap, perfumed ingredients, or other chemical-laden products, you can recommend safer options. See the sidebar Antibacterial Soap: A Dirty Clean (below) for details.

- Avoid synthetic fragrances. Clean babies smell terrific! It bears repeating: synthetic fragrance is really bad for babies. Babies don't sweat and they don't play in mud puddles and your baby routine should reflect the idea that they aren't dirty, so don't be fooled into thinking you need to "perfume" your baby with baby powder, fragranced soaps, or shampoo.

- Try a home remedy. Ask your grandma what she used for nipple pain, diaper rash, or thrush. There are amazing old home remedies that are often quite effective. I've seen parents share such treatments as using baking soda and water for thrush, green tea baths for relieving eczema, and cabbage leaves to cure mastitis. Tell others about those old home-remedies that work for you and try some new DIY recipes of your own.

— green tip —

Antibacterial Soap: A Dirty Clean

In just about every school, childcare facility, and clinic bathroom in North America, you can hear the *splat splat* of antibacterial soap squirting onto the hands of children. Triclosan is the antibacterial ingredient most often used in these soaps. Triclosan is a possible carcinogen, a known endocrine disruptor, is toxic to fish and wildlife, and has been found to increase the risk of antibiotic resistance in humans. Health Canada warns: "These products kill 'good' bacteria, which fight bad germs." Studies show that washing hands with regular soap and water is as effective at killing germs and preventing the spread of infection, and it has fewer scary side effects. The AMA, CMA, and Health Canada all recommend against using antibacterial hand soap.

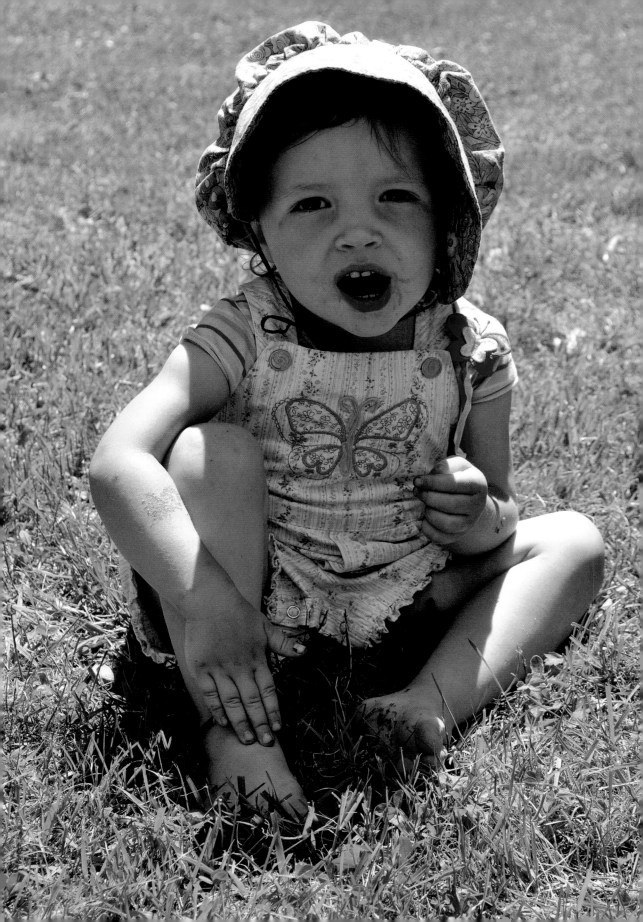

Bare Organics

"It's time to give him a bath," the nurse said to Karen Kerk soon after her son was born. Karen reached into the little bag of hospital freebies and flipped over the little bottle of bath soap to read the ingredients. "Besides water, I didn't know what any of them were: one had 26 letters! The nurse looked at me funny when I decided to just bathe him in plain water instead."

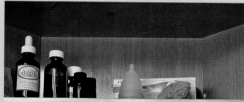

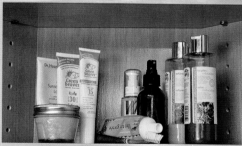

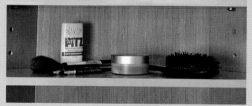

When Karen got home, she searched her local drugstores, grocery stores, and health food spots for something better. "There were lots of choices, but nothing where I recognized all the ingredients." So she did some research, bought a few books and a few good ingredients, and started making products herself. Today, she has a business making the purest skincare products imaginable: Bare Organics. She modelled her company's after the USDA organic standards, relying on organic food-grade ingredients, small batches, and no synthetics.

As much as she loves making products, she loves educating and inspiring parents even more. She answers calls from customers, holds workshops, and teaches classes at the local college. People are especially shocked to learn how bad things are in Canada. "Canadians have this assumption that we are better than the States. But when it comes to skincare, we are a decade behind the States, which is two decades behind Europe."

She advises parents to use fewer products and products with fewer ingredients. Even though she is supposedly in the business of selling personal care products, she still says "Less is more!" with a laugh.

DIY Skincare Recipes for Baby

· ·

Usually, when someone asks me for a recipe, I laugh. A little bit of this and a little bit of that and voila. Thus, all of the recipes below are meant as general suggestions: use what you have on hand, your instincts, and add a bit of love. The better the ingredients (remember, just like you would eat: organic, cold-pressed, unrefined), the better the end product.

Also, remember that essential oils should never be used undiluted on babies because their skin is so porous; however, a few drops added to your baby wipe or bum balm recipe can make a nice-smelling addition that can also help fight infection. Try chamomile, geranium, lavender, lemon, tea tree, rose, rosemary, thyme, or ylang ylang.

Gentle calendula skin oil

A simple oil that can be added to the recipes below or used straight on the baby as a bum barrier, cradle cap salve, or to even help with bruises.

· Dried, organic calendula flowers
· Extra virgin, organic olive oil

Put the dried calendula leaves in a glass jar and pour the olive oil over the leaves so they are completely covered, and then some. Leave the jar in a warm, sunny spot for about 4 weeks or until the olive oil smells like calendula. Strain through cheesecloth. Store in a cool, dark place. It doesn't have preservatives, so it won't last forever.

Bum cream

If you want more of a barrier for your baby's bum than just plain coconut oil, try adding a little shea butter, or experiment with this recipe.

· ½ cup shea butter
· ½ cup coconut oil
· Optional: ¼ cup gentle calendula oil (recipe above; if adding, use ¼ cup less shea butter); 1 tablespoon beeswax; 1 teaspoon zinc oxide powder (for diaper rash–prone babies); a few drops of baby-safe essential oil.

Directions: Melt the shea butter, coconut oil, (optional) beeswax and calendula oil together in a double boiler. Remove from heat once just melted. Do not boil. Add in the (optional) zinc oxide powder. Beat until creamy with an electric mixer, about 8 to 10 minutes. Pour into a jar, stirring in (optional) essential oil drops and let cool.

Baby wipes

Make a little spray bottle for on the go, take your cloth wipes and pre-soak them, or make disposable baby wipes by adding the baby wipe mix to an unbleached, paper towel roll cut in half or a to flushable cloth-diaper liners.

The baby wipe mixture can be as simple as a squirt of Dr. Bronner's, or a similarly gentle castile soap, mixed with a similar size squirt of olive oil into a cup or so of warm water. From there you can add things like aloe vera juice, calendula oil, or a couple of drops of baby-safe essential oils. None of these diaper wipe recipes contain a preservative, so they won't last forever, but they will be good for at least a week. To create solutions that will last a bit longer and fight diaper rash, try adding coconut oil (antimicrobial properties), chamomile tea (mild disinfectant), calendula (mild disinfectant and promotes healing) and/or up to a tablespoonful of raw honey (antibacterial and soothing). If your child has a really bad diaper rash, instead of using more ingredients in your bum cleaning, try just using water at first.

Simple bum wipe recipe

⅛ cup gentle castile soap (like Dr. Bronner's)
⅛ cup edible oil (like extra virgin olive oil)
Few drops of your favourite baby-safe essential oil
2 cups warm, purified water

Simple(ish) bum wipe recipe for diaper rash

2 cups warm chamomile tea (made with purified water)
⅛ cup warm coconut oil
1 tablespoon raw honey, aloe vera gel, or gentle calendula oil
3 drops tea tree oil (optional)
⅛ cup gentle castile soap (optional)
Directions: Combine your ingredients, mix, and then add to your wipes or pour into a spray bottle.

DIY Sunscreen

½ cup olive oil
¼ cup coconut oil
¼ cup beeswax
2 tablespoons shea butter
2 tablespoons zinc oxide (high quality, non-nano)
Optional: a few drops of a non-citrus, baby-friendly essential oil

Directions:

1. In a double boiler (or a jar in a pan of water over low heat) melt the oils, beeswax, and shea butter together.
2. Once melted, remove the mixture from the heat and let cool to room temperature. Whisk in the zinc oxide at this point, being very careful not to breathe in the fumes. You may also add the essential oil at this point, if using.
3. It's ready to use! It isn't waterproof, so reapply often and store in a glass container in the fridge between uses.

TIP: For a shortcut recipe, take your favourite natural skin cream (or your baby's bum balm) and add 2 tablespoons of zinc oxide to that and whip.

Remember, however, that babies less than six months old should never wear any sunscreen, no matter how natural!

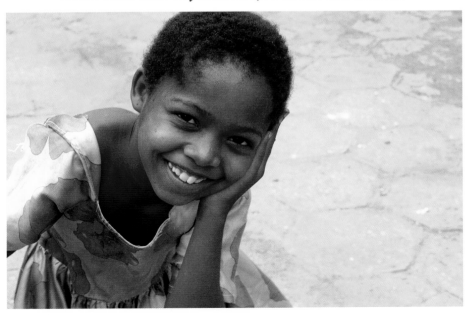

chapter six

Greening Play

· ·

Play is just play. Or is it? Even after having my first child, play equalled toys — beautiful toys that weren't toxic and that would stimulate but not over-stimulate — and managing the inevitable over-accumulation of them. I know, however, from speaking with my grandmother and others of her generation, that play didn't always focus on toys. It was imaginative and free, mostly outside, and rarely supervised — hours and hours of it every day. Toys were rare things. Baby swim classes, toddler gymnastics, and mom-and-me yoga were non-existent.

Scheduled activities aren't the only new inventions: computers, apps, and TV programs designed for babies are also new. These things are fundamentally, and quickly, changing the nature of childhood. Children now attend more classes, have more toys, and are more plugged-in than ever before. It may be hard to guess what this will mean for our children to have imaginative play replaced by toys, screens, and scheduled activities, but there is more research out there about what benefits children and what doesn't than many parents realize. With information, parents can figure out how to walk that increasingly fine line between what is realistic in today's world and what science — and grandma — tells us is best.

Think Like a Scientist of Play

Science tells us that imaginative, unstructured free play is essential and that at least 30 minutes a day of it should be outside. Children do not need a whole bunch of toys to develop well, and more toys may even mean less play. Imaginative play is more educational than any supposedly educational TV program or video game. Secure attachment to parents is the most important element of early childhood development, and use of media by both the parent and child can negatively affect this bond. It is recommended that babies, until the age of at least two, should be shielded from any television or other screens, and even older children benefit from strict limits. And we would all do better and feel better with a bit more fun in our lives (although the organization of your house may suffer!).

The Research

I spoke with dozens of people while researching this chapter — experts, parents, and teachers — and they all made it clear that we can no longer talk about play without talking about technology. When I was young, my family had a tiny black-and-white television: no cable, no tablets or smartphones, and no family computer. We never even considered having a media policy in our household, and though it was a single-parent family where we all ran a little too wild and watched a little too much TV, it never got out of control. How could it with a tiny television set with lines drifting up the screen?

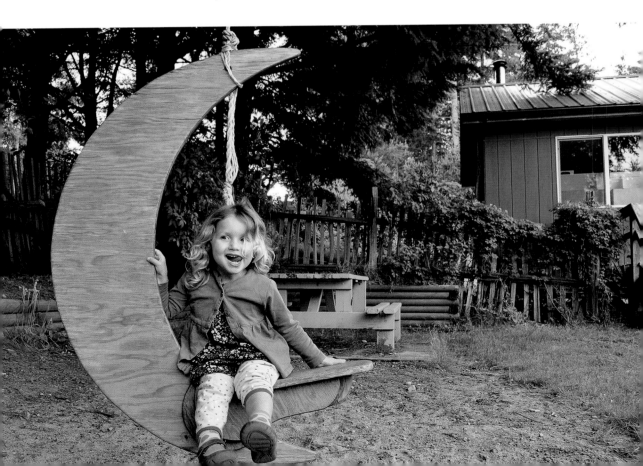

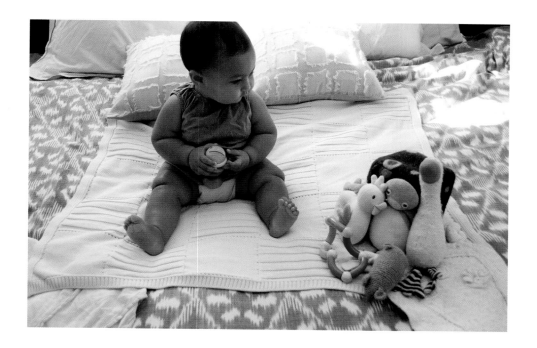

Video games when I was a kid had lots of wires and cartridges for the fun of manipulating a little dot with cursors to avoid other little dots. Looking back now, I think we were lucky that the screens of that time were so *un*compelling. Today, problems arise from too much screen time, too little outdoor time, and not enough free play, especially for children exposed in their early years.

According to Cris Rowan, occupational therapist and author of *Virtual Child: The Terrifying Truth about what Technology Is Doing to Children*, diagnoses of ADHD, autism, motor coordination disorder, sensory processing disorder, self-regulation difficulties (tantrums), aggression, anxiety, depression, and sleep disorders are on the rise. In addition, obesity and mental illness in children are more prevalent today than they were in the past: one in three children enters school developmentally delayed, and one in 11 children between the ages of 8 and 18 is addicted to video games. Causal relationships are hard to prove, but a small peek into Ms. Rowan's research files show correlation between screen time and numerous health problems:

- There is a link between media hours or content and obesity, smoking, sexual behaviour, drug use, alcohol use, low academic achievement, and ADHD according to 80 percent of 173 studies going back to 1980.
- Each hour of TV watched daily between the ages of zero and seven years of age equated to a 10 percent chance of attention problems by age

seven years: three hours a day of TV time equates to a 30 percent greater likelihood.
- Watching television and playing video games are both associated with an increase in subsequent childhood attention problems.
- Every additional hour of TV exposure at 29 months corresponded to a 6 percent decrease in classroom engagement, a 7 percent decrease in math achievement, a 10 percent increase in victimization by classmates, a 13 percent decrease in time spent doing physical activity, and a 10 percent higher consumption of soft drinks and snacks.

Such overwhelming research led pretty much every major health organization, such as the AAP and CPS, to publish guidelines for media use and exposure. According to these organizations:

- Children 0–2 years should have no media exposure (not even background TV);
- Children 3–5 years should have at most one hour per day of tech time; and
- Children 6–18 years should have at most one to two hours per day of tech time.

Furthermore, Ms. Rowan strongly recommends that these times be broken up into 20-minute chunks, beyond which children "zone-out," becoming even more susceptible to the negative impacts. Thus, a five-year-old watching a one-hour video would watch it in 20-minute segments, stop and engage with a person, and then return later for another segment.

A 2010 Kaiser Foundation study shows children now use at least four to five times the recommended media limits: consuming an average of 7.5 hours daily. Even infants are watching an average of two and half hours a day of television. Rowan warns that these numbers are already a few years old and today's numbers are likely higher because of the growing use of tablets and smartphones, with apps designed especially for children.

I know you are desperately hoping right now that this doesn't apply to Baby Einstein, *Sesame Street*, or that Learn-to-Read app you just downloaded. Unfortunately, Rowan says it does: "Parents think that apps, TV programs, and computer programs are educational, but they only entertain. There is no research showing any benefit before grade three, but there is a lot of evidence that shows the negative impact of the early use of tech on kids."

Rowan says that the most important thing for parents to do is to create a healthy foundation for your developing child, just like when you're building a house. In the case of a family, the foundation is a healthy attachment between the parent(s) and the child. She believes that many of the negative consequences from media overuse are actually because media supplants this primary attachment. She encourages parents to begin by examining their own tech use and to consider these guidelines for a balanced approach to media within the family:

- **Who?** Not everyone is the same. Stick to the guidelines above, with lower limits for children with addictions, those with few friends, and those with any of the following conditions: ADHD, obesity, aggression or isolation issues, anxiety, or depression.
- **What?** No violence or sex exposure for those under age 12, and no online gaming until after age 18.
- **When?** Create sacred time where there is no tech distraction allowed at all, such as at dinner, in the car, on holidays, and before bed. You can build these sacred times into the routine of both the day and the year so

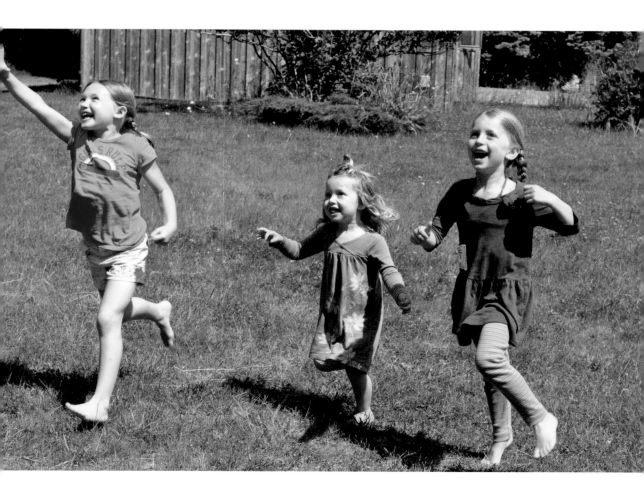

each day there is a no-tech hour, each week a no-tech day, and each year a no-tech week.

- **Where?** Tech time should be social, like the TV time of the 1950s, so it is only used where it can be supervised and shared, such as in high-traffic zones of the house. It should never be used in bedrooms or even cars.

Nature Can Help "Cure" Children

What *doesn't* happen to a child's brain is as important as what *does* happen as they play that video game or are kept quiet thanks to that tablet. Namely, they are not outside engaging in free play. "Young children require three to four hours per day of active rough and tumble play to achieve adequate sensory stimulation to their vestibular, proprioceptive, and tactile systems for normal development," says Rowan.

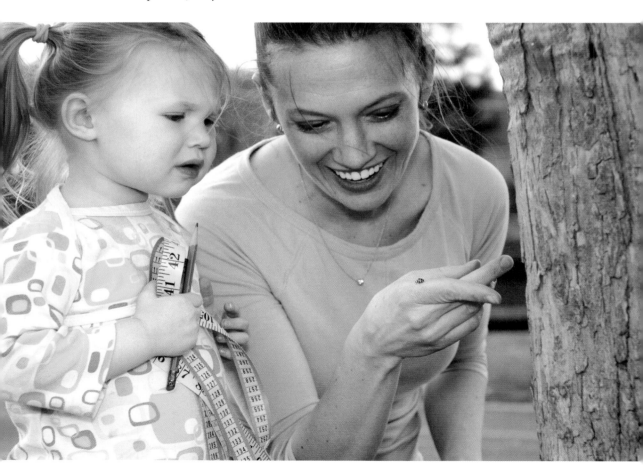

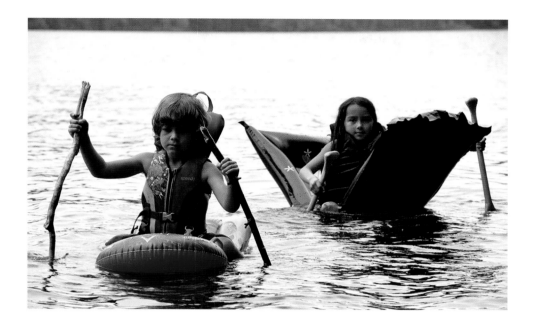

Canadian children get a failing grade when it comes to maintaining a healthy amount of active movement. And in the United States, only a third of high-school-age children get the recommended levels of physical activity according to Let's Move!, an anti-childhood obesity initiative launched by First Lady Michelle Obama. According to Active Healthy Kids Canada, even active video games don't lead to increased overall daily physical activity levels and don't provide the fresh air, connection with nature, and social interactions that come with outdoor play.

Kids aren't getting nearly as much of that outdoor time as they used to. The average North American child spends only half an hour in unstructured outdoor play a day according to the National Wildlife Federation. That's less than half of what it was 20 years ago.

Richard Louv is the award-winning author of *Last Child in the Woods*. His work spawned the "Leave No Child Inside" movement. He says that children's exposure to the natural world improves "health, well-being, and intellectual capacity." As media use increases, our need for nature may actually increase. "The more technology we have, the more nature we need," says Louv. All of these experts — Rowan, Louv, the National Wildlife Federation — discuss the curative potential of outdoor play. Being in nature can reduce ADHD symptoms and stress levels in children and increase test scores. It can even make kids "nicer."

These organizations and experts also point out that lack of physical fitness and outdoor play isn't just the fault of parents, but it's also about our com-

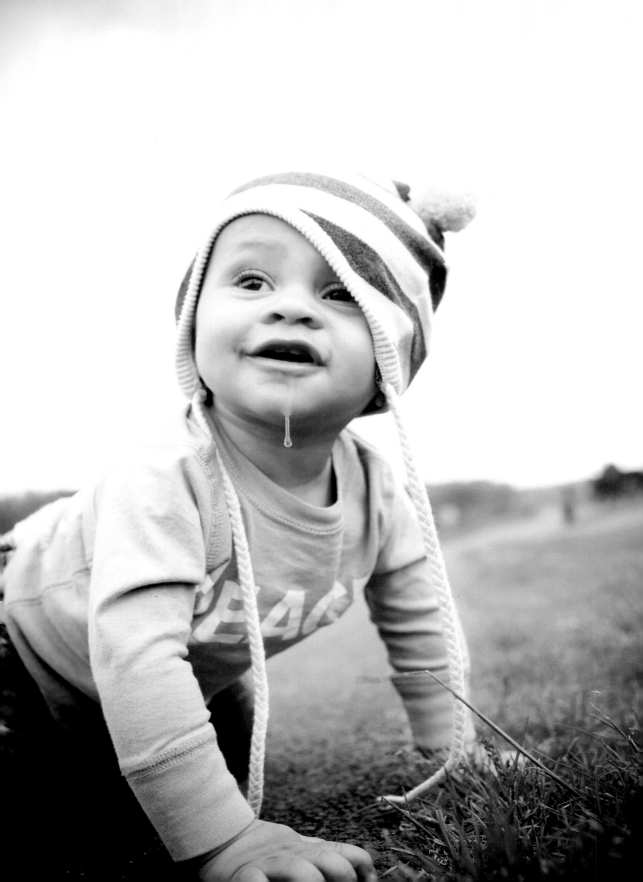

munities, how they are built, and how we can function within them. Healthy neighbourhood design supports fitness as part of daily life. Safe routes for walking and biking to school, natural areas, stimulating playgrounds, and accessible community centres ensure children get the physical activity they need. Louv points out that this is an equity issue. It shouldn't *just* be the children of one ethnic group, class, or even those who have parents who simply value nature more, that get to experience outdoor play. "Every child needs nature," he says.

The Old-Fashioned Analog Toy: Still Toxic?

Play has been an important part of childhood since the founding of North America, according to Howard Chudacoff, author of *Children at Play: An American History*, and that play has gotten increasingly prescriptive, adult-supervised, and laden with toys, media, and other objects, forcing it inside. Perhaps there is no better example of what has happened to American play than the commercialization of toys.

Toys, which once amounted to little more than sticks, spinning tops, and crude baby dolls, have now become a billion-dollar industry. Where once toys were accessories to play, today's toys are often considered to be the play themselves. According to Chudacoff, the more scripted play of today with its specific toys shrinks the size of a child's imaginative space. Playing Barbie with the car and the house or even playing with Lego and putting together a challenging kit is scripted play. A wooden stool that can be turned into a getaway car, become a doll house, or can just be sat on while the escaping princess rests, is a better "toy."

Toys today have other problems besides discouraging creative play. If you, quite reasonably, believe toxins would never be allowed in kids' toys, think again. According to HealthyStuff.org, as many as a third of the most popular children's toys contain toxins. Many of these toys will never be recalled because their chemical components are legal despite known or suspected dangers. Kids' toys don't have their ingredients written in fine print on their labels, so the formaldehyde-laden glue holding together that pressed-wood puzzle, the phthalates in that soft chew toy, and the BPA in those plastic building blocks remain mysteries. And those labels of "non-toxic" or "safe for 0 to 3" don't mean they can't contain known or suspected carcinogens, neurotoxins, or endocrine disruptors.

Many of the thousands of toys that have been recalled over the last few years contained dangerous levels of lead. The element found its way into all sorts of brightly painted children's items, cheap kids' jewellery, and even things like plastic bibs. In 2007, at the height of the "toxic toy" recalls, the *New York Times* reported that 80 percent of toys sold in America were being made in China, where they

"If You Want Your Children to Be Intelligent, Read Them Fairy Tales"

This is a quote from Albert Einstein. And no one knows the truth of this better than Lisabeth and David Sewell McCann, the creators of Sparkle Stories: low-stimulation, warm and gentle stories for children.

As they looked for resources to support their low-media lifestyle, David and Lisabeth realized there was little available. David was a Waldorf teacher and a gifted storyteller, and knew the power of stories to gently guide children. They decided to create and share the transformative power of stories with thousands of listeners. "When you watch screen media it stimulates the lower parts of your brain but shuts down the higher parts.... When you listen to audio stories [the] brain is so busy creating pictures that the children's higher brain is stimulated," explains Lisabeth. "You can tell they are working because afterward the kids get up and play peacefully. After watching television or playing video games, the kids are often agitated."

The importance of storytelling is huge, says child development expert and author Joseph Chilton Pearce. Lisabeth explains why. "When kids are told stories verbally, everything they take in becomes an internal image. They are forever creating the visual world of the story in their mind. It is nourishing for them." After they finish a good story, they come away with "Ahhh, that was so good." They go into a quiet listening space and their brains are busy doing interested, engaged, and relaxed work. Their minds are creating neural pathways. Kids want to hear stories again and again: this is establishing those pathways. In fairy-tales "there is a conflict and there is a beautiful, delightful, funny way to solve it." It helps children internalize these experiences and use them as models in life and to deal with conflict in a peaceful way.

have few safety standards and poor oversight. If lead, a known neurotoxin, can still find its way into kids' products in such astounding numbers, imagine how many other chemicals they may contain, especially those just recently gaining notoriety.

BPA is the perfect example. When the storm of research, media attention, and public outrage struck around the adverse health effects of BPA and the particularly high exposure levels of young children, things changed fast. In 2008, Canada banned the use of BPA in baby bottles, which led the way for other countries to pass similar legislation. This changed the conversation internationally, and many companies voluntarily took BPA off their shelves and out of their products. Some went to alternatives we know are safe, such as glass baby bottles, while others switched to bisphenol S. BPS is very similar in structure to BPA, and studies suggest it also has the ability to disrupt hormone activity even at very low levels.

In *Slow Death by Rubber Duck*, Rick Smith and Bruce Lourie relate similar stories about other substances found in children's toys: vinyl in fashion dolls, phthalates in bath toys, and formaldehyde in rag dolls. A 2011 study published in *Environmental Health Perspectives* found that "most plastic products release estrogenic chemicals." There is no plastic product that has been proven safe for children to mouth or ingest. Parents are catching on: no one can blindly trust that things marketed for children are actually safe for children.

It's Okay to Ditch It All: Free Play Is What Makes Kids Smarter

The information about toys and media is pretty depressing, but the good news is that your children do not need screens or toys to be successful, happy, and smart. Indeed, the key seems to boil down to just one thing: play.

There are seven types of play according to the research of The National Institute of Play. Playing with objects or toys is just one. The other six are:

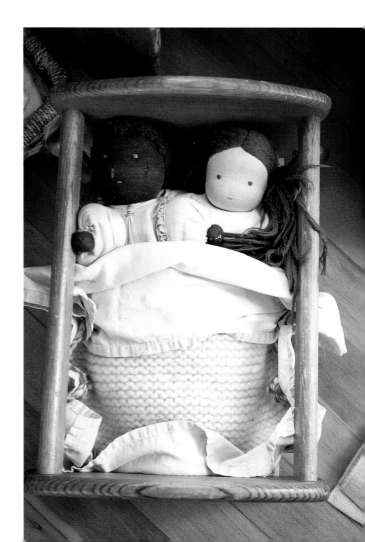

1. **Attunement play** (baby smiles at the mother who smiles back and both feel joy)
2. **Body play and movement** (leaping, swinging, skipping)
3. **Social play** (which includes all kinds of playing together, including parents playing with children)
4. **Imaginative and pretend play** (such as make-believe, fantasy, and other mind play)

5. **Storytelling** (both listening and participating in storytelling)
6. **Transformative-integrative and creative play** (thinking up and making things)

Of all the types of play, make-believe play seems most crucial for young children. It may also be the most at risk of disappearing. Researchers tell us what parents of our current generation already know: many children today do not know how to engage in make-believe play. Some of the reasons are pretty obvious: more television and video games, more soccer and music lessons, and busier parents. Children no longer have the long stretches of unstructured time necessary to get into deep, imaginative play, and they do not have as many opportunities to learn to play from other children, especially older children well-versed in imaginative play.

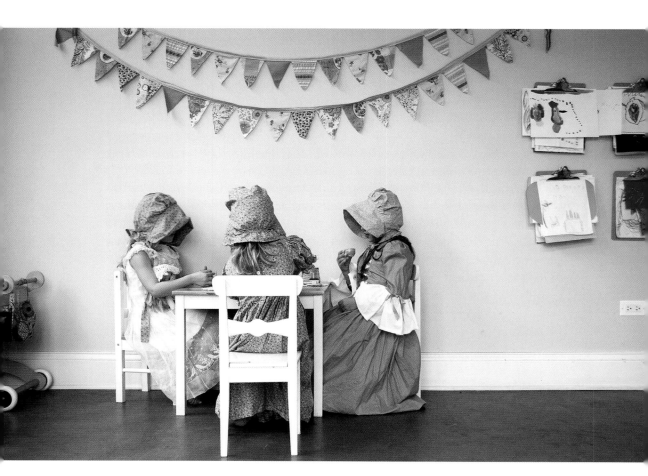

When Money Matters More

While it may seem that not having money would just make it easier to avoid having too many screens, the opposite seems to be true. Let's face it, screens are cheap babysitters and almost everybody has one. Not to mention, there are a lot of people who live in places where it really isn't safe to be outside. I often lived in these very places (although we went outside regardless), but parents today are more likely to keep their kids inside to protect them from the crime and violence prevalent in many neighbourhoods. For things to improve, the conversation needs to change at all levels. Televisions and video games are not acceptable alternatives to affordable childcare and outdoor play. Regardless of financial situation, that is the message we as parents need to spread.

While we wait for government policies to change, affordable childcare is difficult to find. I have joined babysitting co-operatives in which parents take turns watching each other's kids. These can be small arrangements made with a friend or neighbour or larger arrangements like one I was part of in Chicago, where we tracked "hours," needs, and preferences for dozens of families via the Internet.

If you are living on a budget, it is extra important that your child is getting outside every day. I base this in part on my own experience growing up. Too much indoor time puts your child at greater risk of asthma, ADHD, and indoor air pollution exposure. Time in nature can actually counteract some of these problems. If your child is in daycare, find one that prioritizes outdoor time and free-play. Scout out the nearest playground or park to where you live. If it really isn't safe, go to the next closest or look for other pretty outdoor areas.

When I lived in Cleveland, we spent most of our outdoor time exploring the cemetery across the street. No one was ever there and it was beautiful, big, and full of little nooks and crannies to explore. Find a place you can get to as easily as possible from where you live and try to take your child for an hour everyday in all weather. Think of it as a free medicine that is proven to be as effective as drugs for ADHD. It may be good for you as well to spend more time outside. Start when your child is a baby and take the opportunity to walk fast with him in a stroller or in a carrier. Then, let your child crawl and get dirty, and then walk and explore, and so on. Take a book to read instead of your cellphone, or spend the time playing with your child.

Making Less Stuff a Family Value

Maureen Gainer Reilly took her career from helping to organize the homes of the very wealthy to managing projects for large nonprofits that serve the poor. She is also the mother of four young children. In other words, Maureen knows stuff, and she knows how to get it under control. She even knows the key to getting kids to take care of their stuff. "Rich or middle class doesn't matter. Kids now have too many toys. The volume is higher and the quality is lower," she says. Maureen found that the more stuff kids have, the less they play overall and the less they pick up: "Just like when adults get overwhelmed, kids also get overwhelmed with too many choices and too much stuff. If kids have to manipulate or move to get to something they want, they will give up and say they are bored."

Her suggestion is to pare down. "Only keep toys or things that are thought-provoking, such as dress-up, blocks, and Lego," she suggests. She says to never ask your kid if they like a toy: "They like everything!" Instead, say, "Fill this red basket up with your favourites." The rest can go away. They can be donated, re-gifted, or, for the things that parents just can't let go of, they can be packed away in another box to be substituted in or gotten rid of later. She says to use a few big boxes without lids, kept on low shelves, and that are easy for kids to handle. Maybe one could hold blocks, one the dress-up gear picked up at garage sales, and one with all the puppets. It has to be easy for kids if you want them to really play with the stuff and to put it away.

If just thinking about this gives you a panic attack, Maureen can counsel you through that as well. She says wanting lots of stuff is a learned habit, and it can be unlearned as well. She suggests making kids part of the giving away process, but without too many choices.

Maureen directs the conversation of stuff toward the larger question: "What are the values of your family?" She is referring to more than toys and furniture: she is referring to how families spend time and energy. "Just as you control what your kids eat and the amount of TV they watch, I control their experiences and I don't say 'yes' to everything." In particular, she says that she limits the birthday parties, extracurricular activities, and engagements of her family. "These things affect the entire family culture." Evenings and weekends, especially, is family time. "There needs to be down time, time to read, hang out, be bored, make cookies." It's all related, Maureen says, whether it's "with toys, sports, birthday parties, it's important to really ask: 'Is this necessary?'"

Imaginative play helps children develop a critical cognitive skill called executive function, central to the ability to self-regulate. When children can self-regulate they are able to resist impulses, exert self-control, and adapt to varying circumstances. They are capable of starting or stopping their activity, even if they don't want to. Children with good self-regulation abilities can do this even when an adult is not watching, regardless of punishment or reward. "Children who cannot control their emotions at age four are unlikely to be able to follow the teachers' directions at age six," according to researchers at Tools of the Mind. They also say, and other researchers agree, that early development of good executive function, or self-regulation, is a better indicator of school-readiness, and future success in school, than a child's IQ.

Research suggests that children are not self-regulating as well as they used to. A National Public Radio episode on play highlighted an experiment first done in the late 1940s in which researchers had children aged three, five, and seven years

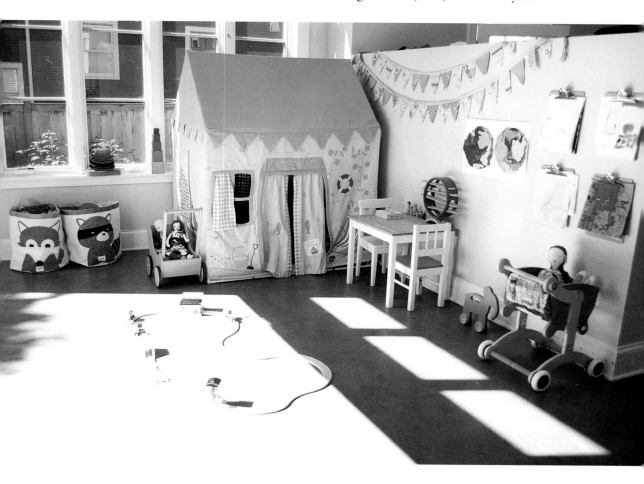

old stand perfectly still without moving. "In the 1940s: the 3-year-olds couldn't stand still at all, the 5-year-olds could do it for about three minutes, and the 7-year-olds could stand pretty much as long as the researchers asked." When they re-created the experiment in 2001, they found that: "Today's 5-year-olds were acting at the level of the 3-year-olds. ... and today's 7-year-olds were barely approaching the level of a 5-year-old."

Just to reiterate, all play is not created equal. Getting outside and doing anything is better than sitting on the couch "playing" video games. The most valuable play is unstructured, imaginative play where kids get to model a level of self-regulation beyond their current level of development. Your child becomes the chef who creates a complicated dinner. He gets other children to set the table, prepare menus, and help serve. Or she becomes a princess needing to escape from an evil witch, develops a plan of escape, and frees the other captives. The potential is endless. The importance is vast. According to Joseph Chilton Pearce, child development expert and author of *The Magical Child* and numerous other books, this kind of play is essential. It is what allows a child to develop the metaphoric, symbolic thinking essential in language, math, science, and in all abstract thought.

Also on the rise today are structured classes, sports for children, and summer camps, none of which have the same level of benefit for children as free, unstructured, imaginative play, according to all these researchers. Indeed, they can severely limit the amount of time a child has for the more important activity of free play in the early years.

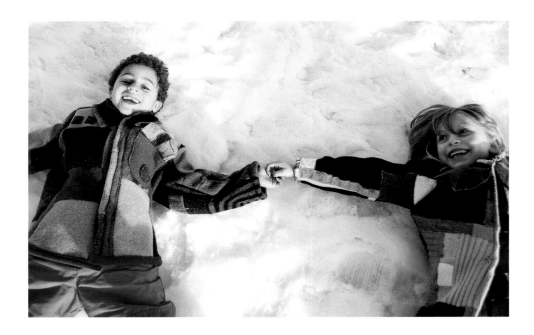

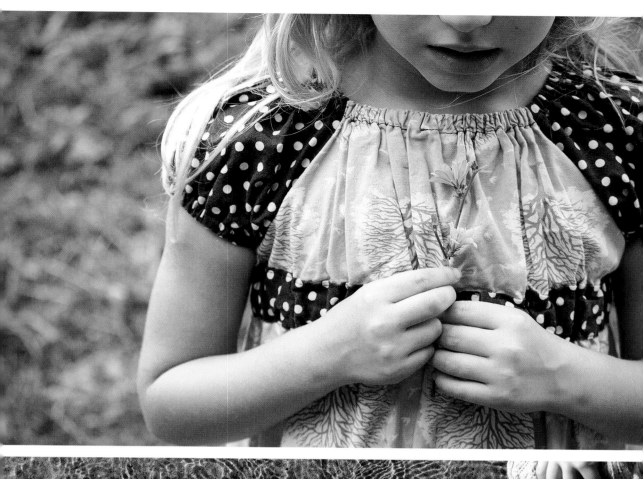
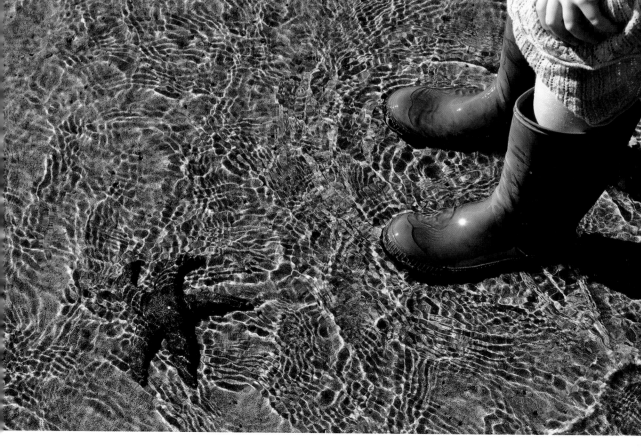

Take Play Seriously

(and Teach Your Kids to Entertain Themselves and Become Smarter, Happier Citizens)

• •

Here are a series of action steps listed from darkest green (biggest impact, possibly more work) to lightest green (quick and easy) to help make healthy play a priority.

- Contemplate the family culture that you want. Do you want your children to play imaginatively together all afternoon, explore the playground alone as they get older, and be happy engaging in family time? These goals lead to concrete decisions and can help give parents the power to say no (it can be awfully hard, can't it?). You now know that children do not benefit as much from structured extracurricular activities as they do from having the time to simply play. Imagine that your first child fulfilled your dream to be a soccer star; your second child became a concert violinist; then imagine this child is your third, and just let her play.

- Build in lots of free time for your child to participate in imaginative play. You don't need to be your child's constant playmate, but you may need to provide guidance. For a young child this can be as simple as showing her how to pretend to drink from an imaginary cup, to make dinner, to wash and hang the laundry, or just about any other daily activity that they see you do. Pretend to be someone else so they get the concept. "Let's pretend we are Papa feeding the baby and putting her to bed." Use simple props like a small baby doll and cups from around the house. Show her how to role play: you can set up the situation for her by saying something like "Papa would say" and then launching right in, talking to the baby, singing, and feeding her. If you have an older child, teach him how to engage his younger siblings with simple roles and help guide the younger child in how to act out these roles.

- Read Maureen's tips on page 138 on how to organize and simplify your stuff. You can get rid of half of it. Go ahead. Start by getting rid of the plastic toys.

- Don't let your baby have exposure to screens. That's right! None. No apps or TV programs are beneficial to young children. The science is extremely clear on this. This means it is also a good time to reflect on your own media use, as children will want to do what they see modelled. Stay as vigilant as you can as long as you can beyond two years. I am here to attest to the fact that your house will seem much messier for a number of years, but one day you will find that your little girl or boy is actually able to disappear into an imaginative world of their own for hours and that there is even space in that imaginative world for younger siblings.

- Don't let your baby chew, gnaw, or mouth on any plastic. No matter how BPA-free it is, plastic is not proven safe: it could contain endocrine disruptors. Just ditch it.
- Safer options for toys and all children products are those time-tested, natural materials such as wool, organic cotton, and wood with safe, food-grade finishes. Now that you know your kids don't need so many toys, you can splurge on getting what you really want. (Maureen has another trick: she returns all the gifts she is ever given for her children and uses the store credits for things her family actually needs.)
- Toys should be open-ended so they can be used by different ages and in different roles. For instance, wood blocks can be stacked and knocked down by a one-year-old and they can be turned into houses for fairies or cars for the five-year-old. Similarly, silk scarves can be a princess dress, a magician's cape, or they can be clipped together to make a tent.
- Avoid toys and art supplies made in China and try to find products made in Canada, the EU, or the United States, where the standards are higher. There is someone near you making beautiful wooden toys. If there isn't, *www.etsy.com* will solve that problem. You can search for recalls in the United States at *www.cpsc.gov* or in Canada at *www.healthy-canadians.gc.ca*.
- Don't buy toys that need batteries. Most parents hate these toys anyway, but the toxic nature of batteries, the inevitable cheap plastic frames, and the lack of imaginative engagement required by the children mean these items are generally bad news.
- Instead of saying "No Gifts" at birthday parties or showers, ask for something specific like a donation to a cause or a contribution toward something you really want like an organic mattress or a new doll house. This method really works!

- Tell stories to your children. Fairytales, especially, can help build a child's imagination and their thinking skills. When you tell stories to young children it is fine to tell the same story over and over; the repetition is healthy for them.
- Help less. Let them navigate more of the playground, park, or living room on their own. One of my first friends to have kids raised his son beautifully with this philosophy: "Lots of little bumps and bruises mean no big ones." And praise them less. The research shows that a child who is often praised will begin to do things for praise rather than for the innate pleasure of doing them. Ultimately, accomplishment is its own reward.
- Petition your local government to make your park appropriate for a variety of children's ages (including older children and even adults). Also, seek out wild places as often as possible and let your child practise climbing trees, navigating rocks, and exploring the woods. Petition your regional and federal government for more assistance to families for childcare and more encouragement for schools to get kids outside.
- Find other parents who are raising their kids with more play. You will find support for your decision to schedule less and give your child the opportunity to play with other kids who know how to play. You can do this as a playgroup, or with individual play dates, or regular family get-togethers, like potlucks.

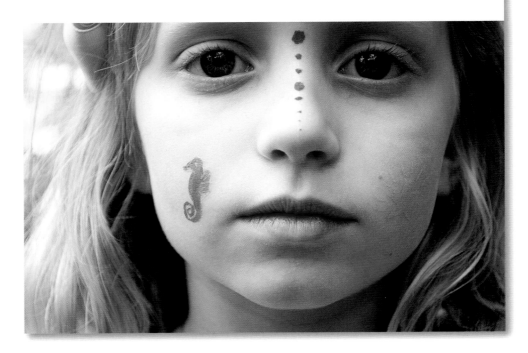

Conclusion

· ·

Now that my children are, in the words of my three-year-old, "Not babies anymore!" the hard work of parenting is just beginning. Establishing a green foundation in the early years helps set the stage for healthier children and gives us parents practice in the tightrope walk of modern parenting — a little bit of grandma's wisdom, a heavy dose of science, and a lot of community support. When I am not sure how to proceed, another trick I practise is to envision the world I want for my child. Then, I work backward to the micro-cosm of my home, family, and womb.

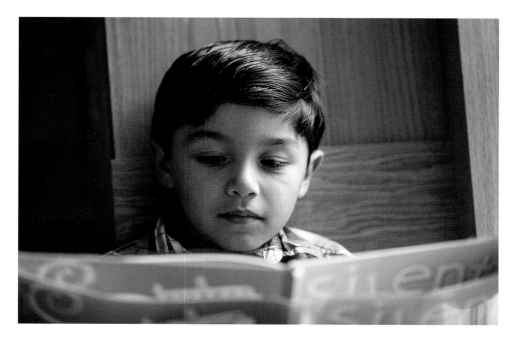

What we do as individuals on one hand matters little. The majority of the world's pollution comes from industry, the majority of the world's inequities come from government policies, and cultural trends are perpetuated on a large scale and enforced by large budgets. Yet, our children are our hope; they are our future. If we believe that our actions change our minds, then we also know that our model will affect our children. Together we are changing minds that will change the world. While on one hand the seed matters little to the tree, it is also everything to the tree. It is the tree's immediate past; it is the tree's impulse to bloom; it is the tree's future.

The principles in this book apply to all aspects of life:

- **Find the answers.** Understand that what you read in the paper, on the Internet, or hear on the news is not the entire story. Do your own research: check out the Resources List and Further Reading sections to get you started. Science works more as a framework for asking question than providing absolute proof. In the meantime, you are the one protecting your child. Ask questions. Stand up to injustice. Demand more from your government.
- **Spend wisely.** Your money is a symbol of your work, your beliefs, and your energy. Spend it on the things that you want more of, things that give you hope.
- **Be willing to go against the trends.** One of my mentors said when she was a new parent she would try to ask what she would do if she were the wild animal version of herself: an ape, wolf, or dolphin. That always seemed

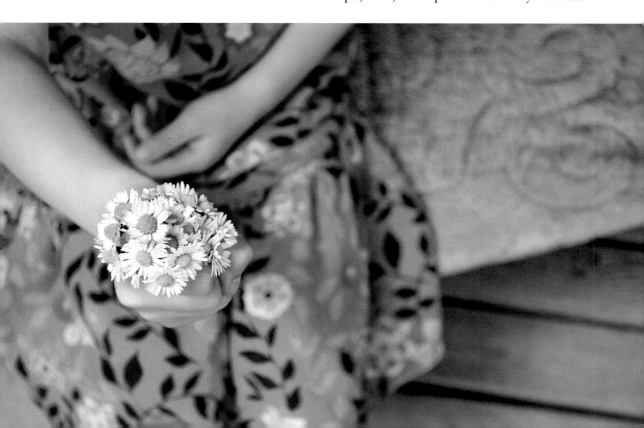

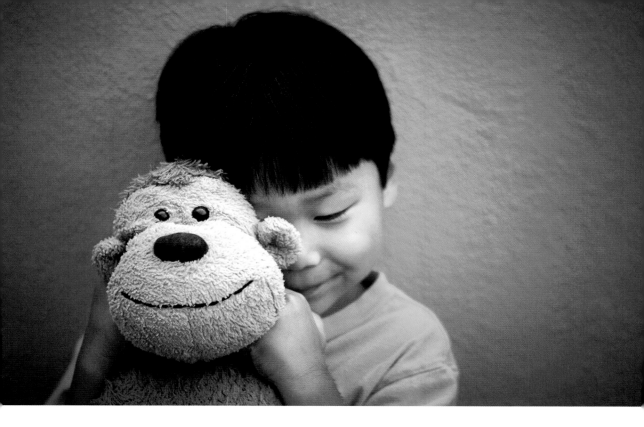

a bit extreme to me, but what has worked for evolution will get you closer to the right path than popular parenting trends. We are designed to protect our children, and we need to expand that to include microscopic and distant dangers as well as ones that are immediate and observable.

- **Get involved globally.** Do not assume "this doesn't apply to me" because you don't live wherever you think the worst things are happening; because of trade and travel, local issues are global issues these days.

- **Do what you love.** There are so many green things to do, so start with the ones that interest you.

- **Create community locally.** Start a playgroup or host a play date. Share green tips, babysitting duties, and meals. It will be easier to stay on your path if you don't feel alone.

- **Be proactive.** Take that minute to write to your representative, to send that email petition, or to make a phone call about the changes you want to see implemented. Politicians act on what they hear their constituents demanding (and sometimes the other "side" is quite loud); companies can change dramatically if they know it matters to their customers. Even if the change you want doesn't happen right away, just doing it makes it easier for you to do it the next time, sets an example for your child, and perhaps on some level it makes it easier for someone else, or many someone elses, to do it too.

- **Play is good for everyone.** Take a moment to skip hand-in-hand with your child, tell each other knock-knock jokes, or go for a hike in the woods or along the beach.

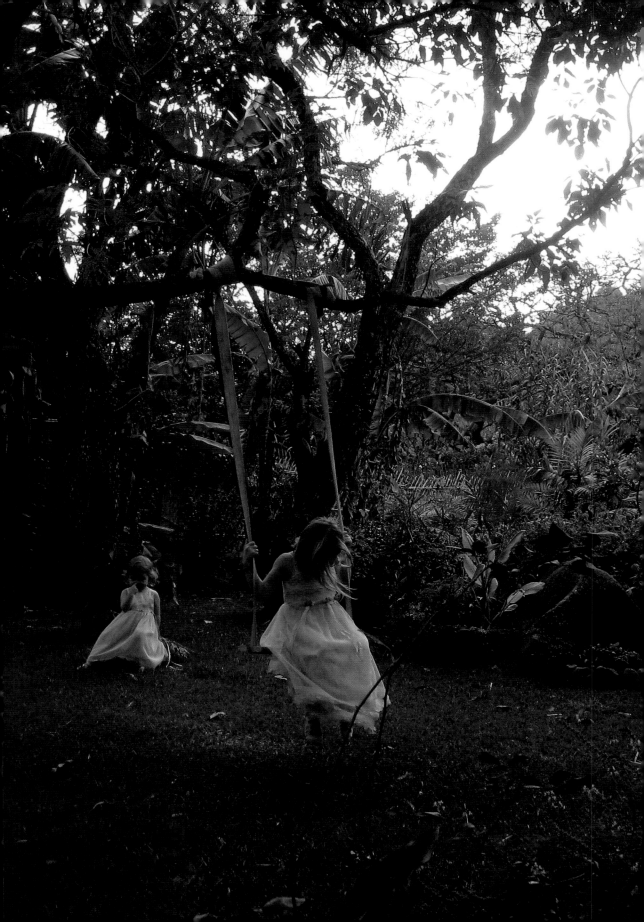

The ABCs of Some Common Toxins

· ·

Formaldehyde

Formaldehyde is a smelly, colourless, flammable gas classified as a Group 1 carcinogen by the IARC. It is known to cause cancer in humans and animals. It can irritate the eyes, nose, and throat, and trigger asthma. Formaldehyde emissions generally decrease over time (i.e. off-gas), but it can take seven years just to reach minimal levels. Unfortunately, the let-it-get-old method of harm reduction doesn't apply to everything that may contain formaldehyde. Old shampoo isn't any safer than the new stuff.

Lead

Lead is a highly toxic heavy metal that persists in the environment and can bioac-cumulate (keeps accumulating in our bodies). Exposure to even a small amount can be hazardous to health. Young children are particularly at risk and during pregnancy it can pass through the placenta to the fetus. Exposure to lead has been linked with hyperactivity, lower IQs, neurocognitive disorders such as ADHD, and it can damage kidneys, blood, muscles, and bones, and is likely carcinogenic. Our lead exposure has decreased thanks to environmental regulations on coal burning, emissions, and the use of lead in consumer products such as paint and gasoline.

Volatile Organic Compounds (VOCs)

VOCs include a wide-range of carbon-based chemicals that easily vaporize (off-gas) from numerous household sources. VOCs can cause immediate health issues, such as headaches, and some have been linked to long-term health effects, including cancer. VOCs react quickly and concentrations will usually decrease over time. Airing new things outside can significantly decrease exposure, but significant amounts can still off-gas from products for many years. Many VOCs have an odour and the "sniff test" can alert you to their presence.

Persistent Organic Pollutants (POPs)

POPs are a major problem for you and your child — and for the polar bears. They remain in the environment and our bodies for a LONG time, perhaps a lifetime. They travel far and like to accumulate in cold places like the polar region — yes, way up there in the "pristine" parts of Canada — where they get stuck. Small amounts can cause big problems, including nausea, learning disabilities, ADHD, autism, thyroid problems, hormonal disruption, and cancer. Most POPs fall into four categories: pesticides, industrial chemicals, brominated flame retardants, and unwanted by-products. Dioxin is a POP, those non-stick substances on your frying pan are POPs, and so are those chemical flame retardants in your child's foam mattress.

Many countries regulate their POPs as part of the 1972 Stockholm Agreement. The original POPs targeted by that agreement, e.g., DDT and Agent Orange, have been substantially reduced in the environment and humans. Unfortunately, we've been developing lots of new POPs.

Chemical Flame Retardants

Some of the most toxic chemical flame retardants are brominated flame retardants (PBDEs) and the phosphate esthers (Tris), including TDCP and TCEP phosphate. PBDEs, TDCP, and TCEP have been linked to serious health problems, including neurological disorders, hormonal disruption, organ damage, thyroid disorders, fertility problems, and may be linked to cancer. Young children are still one of the groups most highly exposed to Tris flame retardants, though they were banned in 1977 from children's sleepwear when they were discovered to mutate children's DNA. PBDE levels are 75 times higher in American women than their European counterparts, likely because of a California law requiring flame retardancy for items sold in that state. Both the United States and Health Canada have asked manufacturers to phase out certain PBDE compounds, but PBDE — as well as Tris — are still on the market and common in children's product. As well, many of the new chemical flame retardants are not much safer.

Dioxin

Dioxin is formed as an unintended by-product of many industrial processes involving chlorine, including the manufacturing of pesticides, the production and incineration of PVC plastics, and paper bleaching. Dioxin was a major ingredient in Agent Orange. Dioxin is often referred to as a super-toxin and the IARC considers the most potent dioxins to be Group 1 carcinogens. They are linked to birth defects, infertility, reduced sperm counts, endometriosis, diabetes, learning disabilities, immune system suppression, lung problems, skin disorders, and numerous cancers. Traces of dioxins can be found in the air, water, and soil, and from there they work their way up the food chain and into fish, animals, and humans. Diet, particular meat and dairy, is considered our primary source of exposure.

Phthalates

Phthalates are found in plastics and cosmetics. They are considered likely hormone-mimickers and have been linked to preterm birth, infertility, and cancer. A CDC study found 75 percent of participants had detectable levels of phthalates in their bodies. The six phthalates considered most hazardous have been banned in the EU since 1999. The United States and Canada have also banned *some* of phthalates in *some* children's products and toys, but not in personal care products.

Toxic Plastics

Plastics are everywhere. They can do amazing things; unfortunately, many, if not most, of them come with some big health costs, including exposing us to chemicals that mimic estrogen. Some of the worst offenders:

- PVC (vinyl) contains lead, phthalates, and releases dioxin. It is linked to neurotoxic effects and endocrine problems. It is found in soft, pliable plastic products like crib mattress covers, bath toys, and, though it is supposed to be banned from them, some teething toys.
- Bisphenol-A (BPA) is one of 39 bisphenol-containing chemicals that are known or suspected endocrine disruptors. BPAs may cause problems of brain and hormone development, decreased sperm counts, erectile dysfunction, heart disease, diabetes, liver abnormalities, and breast cancer. It is found in hard plastic items such as baby bottles and is in the lining of canned goods.

- Melamine is a chemical by-product of industrial processes and is added to some plastics (and some foods, such as in the baby formula scandal). It is linked to kidney failure. Melamine products may also release formaldehyde. It is found in many children's plates and cups that are sold as "BPA-free" or "shatterproof," and looks like hard plastic.
- Polystyrene or Styrofoam contains the toxic substances styrene and benzene, suspected carcinogens and neurotoxins hazardous to humans. Hot foods and liquids, alcohol, oils, acidic foods, and red wine all cause Styrofoam to release toxins into food or drink.

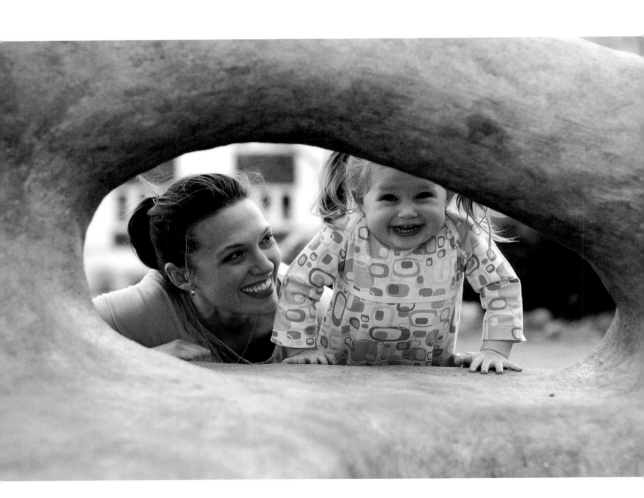

Common Chemicals Found in Children's Personal Care Products

Chemical Name	Health Effects	Products Likely Found In
1, 4-DIOXANE: Look for words ending in "-eth," SLS (sodium laureth sulfate), or PEG	Probable carcinogen	Products that create suds: shampoo, bubble bath, toothpaste, and most baby soap; petroleum-based cosmetics
BORIC ACID, HYDROGEN BORATE	Possible human endocrine disruptor	Baby wipes, baby soap, diaper creams, sunscreen, shampoo, conditioner, skin lotion
IODOPROPYNYL BUTYLCARBAMATE	Potential toxin and neurotoxin. Suspected environmental toxin.	Baby wipes, baby soap, diaper creams, sunscreen, shampoo, conditioner, skin lotion
COAL TAR DYES: COLOUR INDEX (CI) number in Canada or FD&C OR D&C in the U.S., or P-PHENYLENEDIAMINE, NAPHTHA	Coal tar is a known human carcinogen. Artificial food colouring linked to learning disabilities, attention disorders, and hyperactivity in children.	Psoriasis and eczema creams, dandruff shampoo; anything with artificial dyes, including food, hair colour, and makeup

Ethanolamines (MEA, DEA, TEA)	Possible carcinogen	Bubble bath, body wash, shampoo, conditioner, soap, toothpaste
FORMALDEHYDE-releasing preservatives: DMDM HYDANTOIN, DIAZOLIDINYL UREA, HYDROXYMETHYLGLYCINATE, METHANAL, METHYL ALDEHYDE, QUATERNIUM-15	Known human carcinogen	Baby shampoo, conditioner, diaper creams, soaps, lotions, baby wipes
FRAGRANCE/ PERFUME/ PARFUM	May contain known or suspected allergens, carcinogens, neuro-toxins, and endocrine disruptors. Harmful to fish and other wildlife.	Shampoo, conditioner, diaper creams, soaps, lotions, baby wipes (can even be in "unscented" products)
HEAVY METALS, including CALMEL, LEAD ACETATE, MERCURIO, MERCURIC, MERCUROCHROME, THIMEROSOL	Known and suspected neurotoxins and known allergens	Lipstick, mascara, hair dye, deodorant, and can contaminate children's products. Used in some vaccines and topical medications.
OXYBENZONE BENZOPHENONE-3, BENZOYL-5, 5-METHOXYPHENOL, 2-HYDROXY-4-METHOXYBENZOPHENONE-3, METHANONE	Allergen. Forms free radicals to damage skin. Possible endocrine disruptor.	Oxybenzone is the most common ingredient in chemical sunscreens
PARABENS	Suspected endocrine disrupters, reproductive toxins, and neurotox-ins. Links to breast cancer, allergies, and immunotoxicity.	Sunscreen, lotion, soaps, toothpaste, baby oil, bubble bath, shampoo, conditioner

PETROLATUM/ MINERAL OIL/ PETROLEUM JELLY	May be contaminated with polycyclic aromatic hydrocarbons, which may be carcinogenic and possible endocrine disruptors. Inhibit the skin's ability to release toxins.	Baby oils, skin creams, diaper creams, lip balms
PHTHALATES: -phthalate, DBP, DMP, DEP	Possible endocrine disruptors, carcinogens	Found in ¾ of tested products, yet none had phthalates listed on the labels. Avoid products with the words *fragrance*, *perfume*, or *parfum* on their ingredients list.
TOLUENE, 5-DIAMINE, BENZENE	Suspected neurotoxin, endocrine disruptor, and reproductive toxin, known allergen. Harms fish and other wildlife.	Nail polish, nail polish remover, hair dye.
TRICLOSAN (MICROBAN)	Suspected endocrine disrupter. Possible carcinogen. Suspected contributor to antibiotic-resistant bacteria. Harms fish and other wildlife.	Most "antibacterial" products: hand soaps, toothpastes, deodorants, face washes, the lining of gym shoes.

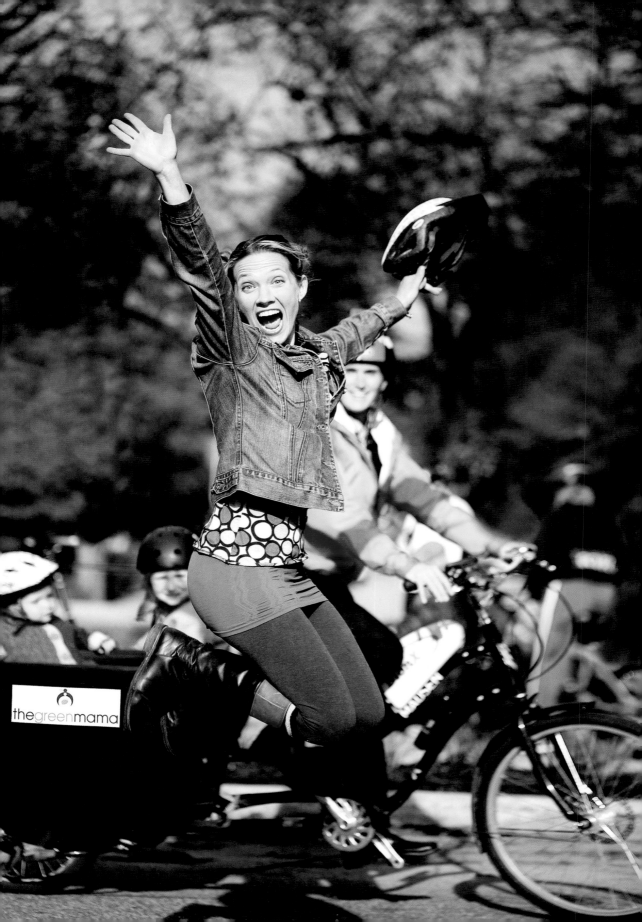

Resources List

· ·

Where can you buy safer, healthier products made by green-minded companies that do well by their employees and the planet? It can be hard, especially for Canadians. There are fewer goods manufactured in Canada than in that land to the south. Many American companies won't ship to Canada (or charge a fortune to do it), and numerous products available in the United States are not legally approved in Canada. Thus, the following list was born. It prioritizes green resources currently available to Canadians and made in Canada.

The risk of naming names is that what's good today may not be good tomorrow, and what's less-than-ideal today just may become better. And, of course, I will inevitably forget some of my favourites (or haven't yet discovered some of the great little companies that deserve recognition). So, always read the labels, please forgive my oversights, and get in touch to let me know what I've missed. You can visit me at *www.TheGreenMama.com* for product reviews and more information on all the subjects covered in this book, or to ask a question.

Cloth Diapering

For help finding cloth diapers made in Canada, visit *etsy.com, canadaclothdiapers. com*, or *dirtydiaperlaundry.com*. To find a hybrid system in Canada, try *grovia. ca* or *gdiapers.ca*. The following are some of the best resources I have found for cloth diapering by province/territory.

Alberta: *adventuresoflittle.ca, bumblebumbaby.com, calgaryclothdiaperdepot.com, clothdiaperkids.com, creationsetcbycandace.ca, diapersupply.ca, happynappy.ca, little-treehugger.ca, pumpkinsdiaperdelivery.com, pureandsimplebabies.ca, rockadrybaby. com, rumparounds.ca, sunbabydiapers.ca, theclothdiapersource.ca, zigglebaby.com*

British Columbia: *bootyboutiqueclothdiapers.com, bumsawaydiapers.com, cozybums. ca, happybabycheeks.ca, hiphuggersdiapers.com, lagoonbaby.com, littlemonkeystore.com, newandgreen.com, shadesofgreenbaby.ca, thebabyfootprint.com, victoriadiaperservice.com*

Manitoba: *ampdiapers.com, howtoclothdiaper.ca*

Newfoundland/Labrador: *glowbugclothdiapers.com/sarah-green*

New Brunswick: *bellybuttonhugs.com, cutiepatooties.net*

Nova Scotia: *bananabottoms.ca, eastcoastdiapers.com, thefluffandstuff-shop.ca, fluffybottombabies.ca, eastcoastdiapers.com, hyenacart.com/stores/ LaPetiteKrottCreations, thecottonpenguin.ca*

Nunavut: Arctic Cotton: *facebook.com/ArcticCotton*

Ontario: *babydue.ca, caterpillarbaby.com, changematt.com, changingwaysdiapers.com, cinnamonbums.ca, cloth-diaper.ca/down-to-earth, clothdiapertrader.com, ellabellabum. com, ecobebeboutique.com, fromthestash.com, funkyfluff.ca, glowbugclothdiapers.com, lilmonkeycheeks.ca, lovepack.ca, minimaestroweb.com, mother-ease.com, naturebumz. com, ottawaclothdiapers.com, snugbugdiapers.com, storkysdiapers.com, theclothdia-pershop.com, tinytreehuggerdiapers.com, trendyecobaby.com, wigglebumsdiapers.ca*

PEI: *bumbleberry.ca, glowbugclothdiapers.com, hautebottoms.com, puddlecatchers.com*

Quebec: *applecheeks.com, amotherstouch.ca, boutiquebummis.com, enfantstylediapers.com, mamanloupsden.com, maiki.com, minikiwi.ca*

Furniture and Accessories

The companies on this list meet the highest standards of design from sustainably harvested woods to food-grade finishes and are made in, or will ship to, Canada. (Currently Health-Canada advises against the use of co-sleepers, so although they aren't forbidden, it is quite hard to find companies that will ship to Canada.)

Austrian Wood Design, The Baby Bunk, Green Cradle, Humanity Organics Family Sleeper, Hushamok, Kalon Studios, Little Merry Fellows Organic Moses basket, Naturalpod, Natarat Juvenile, Pacific Rim, Seed Organic Cradle, Thula, Tulip Juvenile, and Vermont Woods Studio.

Mattresses, Bedding, Nursing Pillows, and Puddle Pads

Aviva, Dream Designs, Essentia, Grass Roots, Green Sleep, Hastens, inBed Organics, Kushies, The Mattress and Sleep Company, Mayukori, Natura, Nneka, Obasan/Sleeptek, Organic Lifestyle, Organic Quilt Company, Rawganique, Royal-Pedic, Shepherd's Dream, St. Geneve, and Thula.

Pajamas, Sleep Sacks, and Swaddles

The Dream Bag, ergoPouch, Green Bean Baby, Innocent Earth, Kohlr Baby, Kushies, Lulujo, Made in Heaven, Mini Mioche, Nosilla Organics, Om Home, Parade Baby, Tree House Funwear, Wee Urban Baby, Wee Woolies, Woolino.

Skincare

Aleva Naturals (*alevanaturals.com*), All Things Jill (*allthingsjill.ca*), Bare Organics (*bareorganics.ca*), Carré Jaune (*carrejaune.ca*), Dimpleskins Naturals (*dimpleskinsnaturals.com*), Green Beaver (*www.greenbeaver.com*).

Other Online Baby Care Retailers (by Province)

Alberta: *babesinarms.ca*, *clothdiaperkids.com*, *naturesbabybasket.com*, *rivasecostore. com*, *turtlesinbloom.com* (Calgary), *sashabeanbaby.ca*, *tinyfootprinttoys.ca* (Edmonton), *blankiesandbums.ca* (Fort McMurray) *ecobabycanada.com* (Lethbridge)

British Columbia: *abbysprouts.com*, *goodplanet.com* (Victoria), *huckleberry-babyshop.com*, *lalaladybug.com* (Nanaimo), *kradles.ca*, *podlings.ca* (Courtenay), *crocodilebaby.com greenbeanbaby.com*, *hipbaby.com*, *lavishandlive.com*, *lilwonders. ca*, *littleearthvancouver.com*, *mylittlegreenshop.com*, *organicallyhatched.com*, *raspberrykids.com* (Vancouver), *lussobaby.ca* (North Vancouver), *lizziebaby.ca* (Kamloops), *thegreensheep.ca* (Prince George), *thespottedowl.ca* (Duncan)

Manitoba: *babygreensprout.com*, *tinytreehuggerdiapers.com* (Niverville), *www. etsy.com/shop/SweetSparrowDesign* (Winkler)

Newfoundland/Labrador: *belliesandbundles.ca*, *flowerchildonline.com* (St. John's)

New Brunswick: *a-little-something-for-everyone.com* (Upper Coverdale), *ana-bananababy.com* (Moncton)

Nova Scotia: *goasyougrow.ca* (New Minas), *enchanted-forest.ca* (Truro), *plovers. net* (Halifax), *blackvioletbaby.com* (Berwick)

Ontario: *babycharlotte.com* (Kitchener), *advicefromacaterpillar.ca*, *avasappletree. ca*, *babygreensprout.ca*, *babyonthehip.ca*, *babyorganicjoy.ca*, *ecoexistence.ca*, *kaikids. com*, *organiclifestyle.com*, *the100mildchild.ca* (Toronto), *bynature.ca* (Orillia), *barefootbabies.ca*, *citizenkid.ca* (Hamilton), *ecobebeboutique.com* (Ottawa), *go-greenbaby.ca* (Kingston), *jesscrunchyshop.com* (Kitchener), *littlelamb.ca* (Timmins) *happybumz.com* (Cobourg) *snugglebugz.ca* (Burlington)

PEI: *greenwithjoy.ca*

Saskatchewan: *babyluvboutique.com* (Humboldt), *mothersmelody.ca* (Saskatoon)

Yukon: *duenorthmaternityandbaby.com*

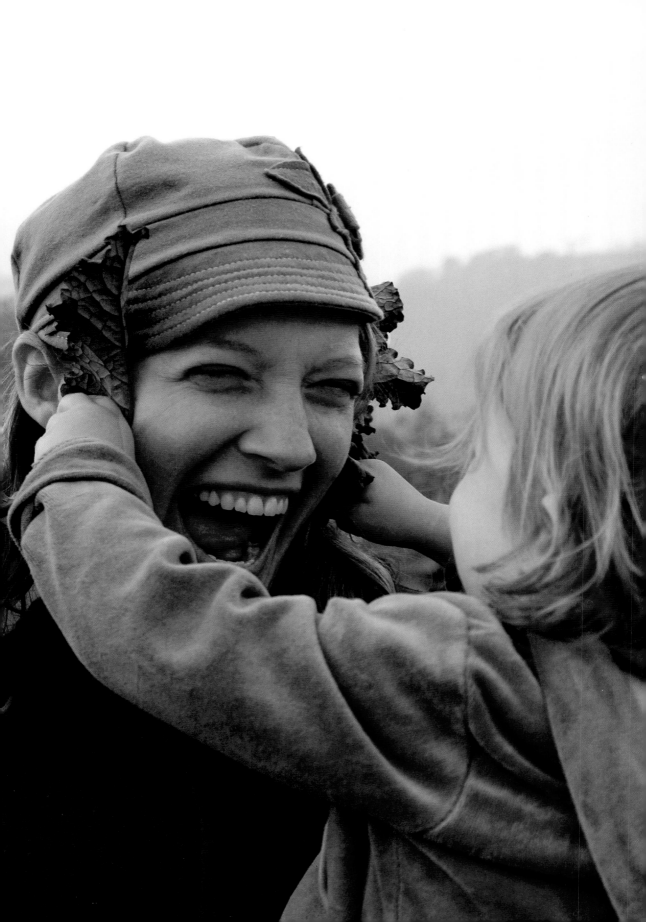

Further Reading

Books

Maria Armstrong and Shell Walker, *Resources for Informed Breastmilk Sharing*

Rahima Baldwin Dancy, *You Are Your Child's First Teacher: Encouraging Your Child's Natural Development from Birth to Age Six*

Ingrid Bauer, *Diaper Free: The Gentle Wisdom of Natural Infant Hygiene*

Jennifer Block, *Pushed: The Painful Truth about Childbirth and Modern Maternity Care*

Laurie Boucke, *Infant Potty Training*

Robert Bradley and Ashley Montagu, *Husband Coached Childbirth: The Bradley Method of Natural Childbirth*

Heidi Britz-Crecelius, *Children at Play: Using Waldorf Principles to Foster Childhood Development*

Po Bronson and Ashley Merryman, *NurtureShock: New Thinking about Children*

Rachel Carson, *Silent Spring*

Joseph Chilton Pearce, Magical Child series

Howard Chudacoff, *Children at Play: An American History*

Shea Darian, *Seven Times the Sun: Guiding Your Child Through the Rhythms of the Day*

Gillian Deacon, *There's Lead in Your Lipstick*

Heather Dessinger, *Nourished Baby*

Kelly Dorfman, *Cure Your Child with Food*

Pam England, *Birthing from Within: An Extra-Ordinary Guide to Childbirth*

Sally Fallon, *Nourishing Traditions*

Margaret Floyd Barry, Eat Naked series

Selma Fraiberg, *The Magic Years*

Ina May Gaskin, *Ina May's Guide to Breastfeeding; Ina May's Guide to Childbirth*

Machaela Glockler and Wolfgang Goebel, *A Guide to Child Health: A Holistic Approach to Raising Healthy Children*

Henci Goer, *The Thinking Woman's Guide to a Better Birth*

Tracy Hogg and Melinda Blau, *Secrets of the Baby Whisperer: How to Calm, Connect, and Communicate with Your Baby*

Kathleen Huggins, *The Nursing Mother's Companion*

Harvey Karp, *The Happiest Baby on the Block: The New Way to Calm Crying and Help Your Newborn Sleep Longer*

La Leche League International, *The Womanly Art of Breastfeeding*

Karen Le Billon, *French Kids Eat Everything & So Can Yours*

Jill Lekovic, *Diaper Free Before 3: The Healthier Way to Toilet-Train and Help Your Child Out of Diapers Sooner*

Dr. Nicole Letourneau and Justin Joschko, *Scientific Parenting: What Science Reveals about Parental Influence*

Alicia F. Lieberman, *The Emotional Life of the Toddler*

Jean Liedloff, *The Continuum Concept: In Search Of Happiness Lost*

Bruce Lourie and Rick Smith, *Slow Death by Rubber Duck: How the Toxic Chemistry of Everyday Life Affects Our Health; Toxin Toxout: Getting Harmful Chemicals Out of Our Bodies and Our World*

Richard Louv, *Last Child in the Woods: Saving Our Children from Nature-Deficit Disorder*

Larry Malerba, *Green Medicine: Challenging the Assumptions of Conventional Health Care*

Susan Markel, *What Your Pediatrician Doesn't Know Can Hurt Your Child*

Gordon Neufeld and Gabor Maté, *Hold On to Your Kids: Why Parents Need to Matter More Than Peers*

Kim John Payne and Lisa M. Ross, *Simplicity Parenting*

Nina Planck, *Real Food for Mother and Baby: The Fertility Diet, Eating for Two, and Baby's First Foods*

Michael Pollan, *The Omnivore's Dilemma: A Natural History of Four Meals*

Aviva Jill Romm, *Vaccinations: A Thoughtful Parent's Guide*

Amanda Rose, *Rebuilding from Depression*

John Rosemond, *The Well-Behaved Child: Discipline that Really Works*

Cris Rowan, *Virtual Child: The Terrifying Truth about What Technology Is Doing to Children*

Robert Sears, *The Vaccine Book: Making the Right Decision for Your Child*

William Sears, *The Baby Book: Everything You Need to Know about Your Baby*

Daniel Siegel and Tina Payne Bryson, *The Whole-Brain Child*

Meredith Small, *Our Babies, Ourselves*

Sandra Steingraber, *Having Faith: An Ecologist's Journey to Motherhood; Raising*

Elijah: Protecting Our Children in an Age of Environmental Crisis

Annemarie Tempelman Klut, *Healthy Mum, Happy Baby: How to Feed Yourself When You're Breastfeeding Your Baby*

Adria Vasil, Ecoholic series

Marc Weissbluth, *Healthy Sleep Habits, Happy Child*

Kelly Wels, *Changing Diapers: The Hip Mom's Guide to Modern Cloth Diapering*

Toni Weschler, *Taking Charge of Your Fertility: The Definitive Guide to Natural Birth Control, Pregnancy Achievement, and Reproductive Health*

Websites

activehealthykids.ca
activekidsclub.com
BestForBabes.org
BFMed.org
bornready.co.uk
BreastFeedingCanada.ca
BreastFeedingInc.ca
CanadianBreastfeedingFoundation.org
cape.ca
cbf.org/ncl
cec.org
chehc.ca
childrenandnature.org
childrensenvironment.ca
cich.ca
cornucopia.org
davidsuzuki.org
diaperfreebaby.org
eartheasy.com
EatsonFeets.org
ecoparent.ca
ecsimplified.com
ecwear.com
ewg.org
healthandenvironment.org
healthtoys.org
healthychild.org

healthyenvironmentforkids.ca
healthystuff.org
InFactCanada.ca
infantrisk.com
KellyMom.com
letsmove.gov
llli.ca
llli.org
mothering.com
motherisk.org
nrdc.org
organicconsumers.org
parttimeec.com
realdiaperassociation.org
safecosmetics.org
silentspring.org
TheLeakyBoob.com
toolsofthemind.org
toxicfreecanada.ca
toxnet.nlm.nih.gov
tribalbaby.org
wen.org.uk
westonaprice.org
whatsonmyfood.org
whywaldorfworks.org
wilderness.org
womensvoices.org

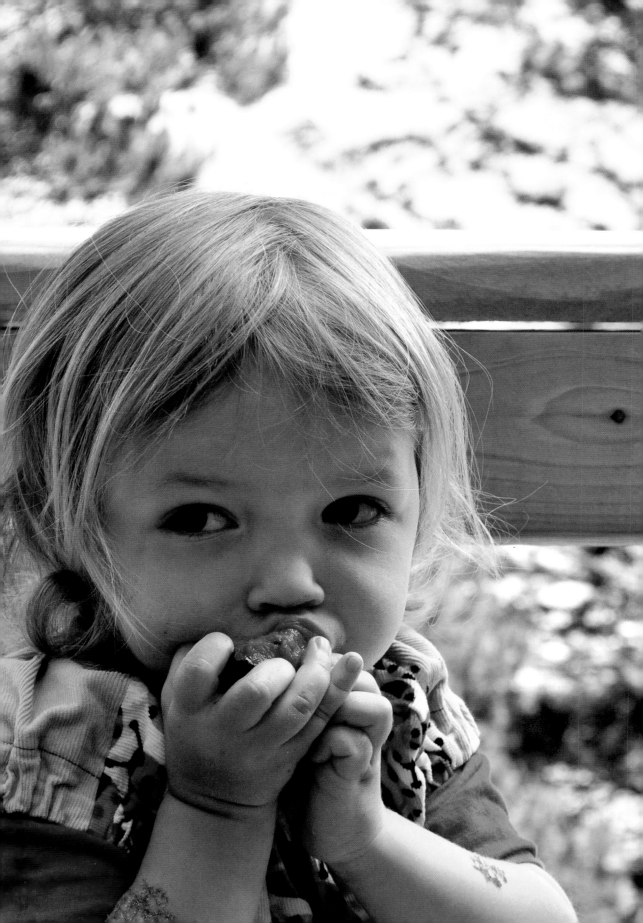

Sources

Introduction (and Appendices)

"Asthma Rates in Children Have Jumped Fourfold: Report." *CBC News*, January 27, 2006.

Autism Speaks Canada. "Facts and Stats." March 2012.

Bushnik, Tracey, Jocelynn L. Cook, A. Albert Yuzpe, Suzanne Tough, and John Collins. "Estimating the Prevalence of Infertility in Canada." *Human Reproduction* 27, no. 3 (2012): 738–46. doi:10.1093/humrep/der465.

Canadian Diabetes Association. "Children and Type 2 Diabetes." *www.diabetes.ca/diabetes-and-you/youth/type2.*

Canadian Mental Health Association. "Fast Facts about Mental Illness." *www.cmha.ca/media/facts-about-mental-illness.*

Carlsen, E., A. Giwercman, N. Keiding, and N.E. Skakkebaek. "Evidence for Decreasing Quality of Semen During Past 50 Years." *BMJ* 305, no. 6854 (1992): 609–13.

CDC. "Asthma: Data and Surveillance." March 25, 2013. *www.cdc.gov/asthma/asthmadata.htm.*

———. "National Diabetes Fact Sheet: National Estimates and General Information on Diabetes and Prediabetes in the United States, 2011." Atlanta, GA: U.S. Department of Health and Human Services.

Childhood Obesity Foundation. "Statistics." *www.childhoodobesityfoundation.ca/statistics.*

Connor, Steve. "Out for the Count: Why Levels of Sperm in Men Are Falling." *The Independent*, December 1, 2013.

EWG and Commonweal. "Human Toxome Project: Mapping the Pollution in People." 2014.

Ferguson, K.K., T.F. McElrath, and J.D. Meeker. "Environmental Phthalate Exposure and Preterm Birth." *JAMA Pediatrics* 168, no. 1 (2014): 61–67. doi:10.1001/jamapediatrics.2013.3699.

Harris, Pam. "Mental Illness on the Rise in America's Children." *Medscape.* May 16, 2013.

Kinsley, Howard Craig Meyer, and Elizabeth Meyer. "Maternal Mentality." *Scientific American Mind*, July 2011: 22.

Laurance, Jeremy. "Scientists Warn of Sperm Count Crisis." *The Independent*, December 1, 2013.

Lip, S.Z.L., Louise Murchison, Paul Cullis, Lindsay Govan, and Robert Carachi. "A Meta-Analysis of the Risk of Boys with Isolated Cryptorchidism Developing Testicular Cancer in Later Life." *Archives of Disease in Childhood* 98, no. 1 (2012): 20–26. doi:10.1136/archdischild-2012-302051.

Mossop, Brian. "The Science of Fatherhood." *Scientific American Mind*, July 2011: 24–30.

National Cancer Institute. "Fact Sheet: Childhood Cancers." *www.cancer.gov/cancertopics/factsheet/Sites-Types/childhood*.

Pittman, Genevra. "Almost One in Six Couples Face Infertility: Study." *Reuters* (U.S. edition), January 11, 2013. *www.reuters.com/article/2013/01/11/us-couples-infertility-idUSBRE90A13Y20130111*.

President's Cancer Panel. "Reducing Environmental Cancer Risk: What We Can Do Now." 2008–2009 Annual Report, 2010.

Schapiro, Mark. "Toxic Inaction: Why Poisonous, Unregulated Chemicals End Up in Our Blood." *Harper's Magazine*, October 2007.

Siegel, Daniel. "The Neurological Basis of Behavior, the Mind, the Brain, and Human Relationships." Talk at the Climate, Mind, and Behavior Symposium, Garrison Institute, New York, 2011.

Skakkebaek, N.E., E. Rajpert-De Meyts, and K.M. Main. "Testicular Dysgenesis Syndrome: An Increasingly Common Developmental Disorder with Environmental Aspects: Opinion." *Human Reproduction* 16, no. 5 (2001): 972–78. doi:10.1093/humrep/16.5.972.

Smith, Rick, and Bruce Lourie. *Slow Death by Rubber Duck: How the Toxic Chemistry of Everyday Life Affects Our Health*. Toronto: Random House, 2009.

Stobbe, Mike. "More Than One in 10 Children Diagnosed with ADHD as Rates of Disorder Rise in U.S.: Survey." *National Post*, November 22, 2013.

Swan, S.H., E.P. Elkin, and L. Fenster. "Have Sperm Densities Declined? A Reanalysis of Global Trend Data." *Environmental Health Perspectives* 105, no. 11 (1997): 1228–232.

————. "The Question of Declining Sperm Density Revisited: An Analysis of 101 Studies Published 1934–1996." *Environmental Health Perspectives* 108, no. 10 (2000): 961–66.

Thoma, Marie E., Alexander C. McLain, Jean Fredo Louis, Rosalind B. King, Ann C. Trumble, Rajeshwari Sundaram, and Germaine M. Buck Louis. "Prevalence of Infertility in the United States as Estimated by the Current Duration Approach and a Traditional Constructed Approach." *Fertility and Sterility* 99, no. 5 (2013): 1324–331.

Tremonti, Anna Maria. "Diagnosing ADHD: Are We Getting It Right?" *The Current*, CBC, April 9, 2013.

Völkela, W., O. Genzel-Boroviczényb, H. Demmelmairb, et al. "Perfluorooctane Sulphonate (PFOS) and Perfluorooctanoic Acid (PFOA) in Human Breast Milk: Results of a Pilot Study." *International Journal of Hygiene and Environmental Health* 211, nos. 3–4 (2008): 440–46.

Greening the Nursery and Home

Arizona Department of Environmental Quality. "Children Are Not Little Adults." *www.azdeq.gov/ceh/risks.html*.

BC Centre for Disease Control, National Collaborating Centre for Environmental Health. "Radiofrequency Toolkit for Environmental Health Practitioners." 2013.

Buffer, Janet, Lydia Medeiros, Mary Schroeder, Patricia Kendall, Jeff LeJeune, and John Sofos. "Cleaning and Sanitizing the Kitchen Using Inexpensive Household Food-Safe Products." The Ohio State University, revised 2010.

CDC. "Guideline for Disinfection and Sterilization in Healthcare Facilities." 2008.

Environmental Protection Agency. "An Introduction to Indoor Air Quality." *www.epa.gov/iaq/ia-intro.html.*
——— "Questions about Your Community: Indoor Air." *www.epa.gov/region1/communities/indoorair.html.*

Gibson, Rachel, and Travis Madsen. "Toxic Baby Furniture: The Latest Case for Making Products Safe from the Start." Environment California Research and Policy Center, May 2008.

Gilling, D.H., M. Kitajima, J.R. Torrey, and K.R. Bright. Antiviral Efficacy and Mechanisms of Action of Oregano Essential Oil and Its Primary Component Carvacrol Against Murine Norovirus. *Journal of Applied Microbiology* (published online first) February 12, 2014. doi:10.1111/jam.12453.

International Agency for Research on Cancer (June 2004). IARC Monographs on the Evaluation of Carcinogenic Risks to Humans Volume 88 (2006): Formaldehyde, 2-Butoxyethanol and 1-tert-Butoxypropan-2-ol.

Lebowitz, Michael. "Asthma Increasingly Affecting North American Children." Commission for Environmental Cooperation, Summer 2001.

McGwin, Gerald, Jeffrey Lienert, and John I. Kennedy, Jr. "Formaldehyde Exposure and Asthma in Children: A Systematic Review." *Environmental Health Perspectives* 118, no. 3 (2010): 313–17.

Mott, Lawrie, David Fore, Jennifer Curtis, and Gina Solomon. "Our Children At Risk: The Five Worst Environmental Threats to Their Health." National Resource Defence Council, November 1997.

Moyers, Bill, and Judit Davidson Moyers. *Trade Secrets: A Moyers Report.* PBS. Public Affairs Television, Inc., 2001.

National Institutes of Health: National Cancer Institute. "Fact Sheet: Formaldehyde and Cancer." *www.cancer.gov/cancertopics/factsheet/Risk/formaldehyde.*

Olson, David A., and Richard L. Corsi. "In-Home Formation and Emissions of Trihalomethanes: The Role of Residential Dishwashers." *Journal of Exposure Science and Environmental Epidemiology* 14 (2004): 109–19. doi:10.1038/sj.jea.7500295.

Royce, S., and H. Needleman. "Case Studies in Environmental Medicine: Lead Toxicity." Agency for Toxic Substances and Disease Registry, 1995.

Stapleton, Heather M., Susan Klosterhaus, Alex Keller, et al. "Identification of Flame Retardants in Polyurethane Foam Collected from Baby Products." *Environmental Science and Technology* 45, no. 12 (2011): 5323–331. doi:10.1021/es2007462.

U.S. Environmental Protection Agency, Office of Air and Radiation. *Report to Congress on Indoor Air Quality* Volume II. *Assessment and Control of Indoor Air Pollution.* 1989.

Zekert, Ashley E., "Effect of Alternative Household Sanitizing Formulations Including: Tea Tree Oil, Borax, and

Vinegar, to Inactivate Foodborne Pathogens on Food Contact Surfaces." Thesis, Virginia Polytechnic Institute and State University, 2009.

Greening the Bum

Allsop, Michelle. "Achieving Zero Dioxin." London: Greenpeace International, 1994.

Anderson, Rosalind, and Julius Anderson. "Acute Respiratory Effects of Diaper Emissions." *Archives of Environmental Health* 54, no. 5 (1999): 353–58. doi:10.1080/00039899909602500.

Bakker, E., J.D. Van Gool, M. Van Sprundel, C. Van Der Auwera, and J.J. Wyndaele. "Results of a Questionnaire Evaluating the Effects of Different Methods of Toilet Training on Achieving Bladder Control." *BJU International* 90, no. 4 (2002): 456–61.

Barone J.G., N. Jasutkar, and D. Schneider. "Later Toilet Training Is Associated with Urge Incontinence in Children." *Journal of Pediatric Urology* 5, no. 6 (2009): 458–61.

Blum, Nathan, Bruce Taubman, and Nicole Nemeth. "Relationship Between Age at Initiation of Toilet Training and Duration of Training: A Prospective Study." *Pediatrics* 111, no. 4 (2003): 810–14.

Environmental Health Association of Nova Scotia. *The Guide to Less Toxic Products. www.lesstoxicguide.ca*.

Goode, Erica. "Two Experts Do Battle Over Potty Training." *New York Times*, January 12, 1999.

Greenpeace. "New Tests Confirm TBT Poison in Procter & Gamble's Pampers: Greenpeace Demands World-Wide Ban of Organotins in All Products." May 15, 2000.

Gupta, A.K., and A.R. Skinner. "Management of Diaper Dermatitis." *International Journal of Dermatology* 43, no. 11 (2004): 830–34. doi:10.1111/j.1365-4632.2004.02405.x.

Largo, R.H., K. von Siebenthal, and U. Wolfensberger. "Does a Profound Change in Toilet-Training Affect Development of Bowel and Bladder Control?" *Developmental Medicine & Child Neurology* 38, no. 12 (1996): 1106–116.

Lehrburger C., J. Mullen, and C.V. Jones. "Diapers: Environmental Impacts and Lifecycle Analysis." Philadelphia, PA: The National Association of Diaper Services (NADS), 1991.

Milieu Centraal. "Dutch Study on Environmental Impacts of Cloth Versus Disposable Diapers." April 22, 2008. *www.milieucentraal.nl/thema%27s/thema-2/artikelen-kopen-en-gebruiken/luiers/*. Translated version: *www.twinkleontheweb.co.uk/DutchNappyReport.html*.

Mullen, Angelique. "Diaper Rash: Comparing Diaper Choices." *Real Diaper News*, August 2005. Real Diaper Association.

Partsch, C.J., M. Aukamp, and W.G. Sippell. "Scrotal Temperature Is Increased in Disposable, Plastic Lined Nappies." *Archives of Disease in Childhood* 83, no. 4 (2000): 364–68. doi:10.1136/adc.83.4.364.

Stein, Howard. "Incidence of Diaper Rash When Using Cloth and Disposable Diapers." *The Journal of Pediatrics* 101, no. 5 (1982): 721–23.

UK Environment Agency. "Using Science to Create a Better Place: An Updated Lifecycle Assessment Study for Disposable and Reusable Nappies." SC010018/SR2. 2008.

Women's Environmental Network. "Environment Agency Nappy Report Is Seriously Flawed." 2005. Media Release.

Greening the Boobs

American Academy of Pediatrics. "Breastfeeding and the Use of Human Milk." *Pediatrics* 115, no. 2 (2005): 496–506.

Armstrong, M., and S. Walker. "Resource for Informed Breastmilk Sharing." *www.eatsonfeetsresources.org*.

Ball, T.M., and A.L. Wright. "Health Care Costs of Formula-Feeding in the First Year of Life." *Pediatrics* 103, no. 4.2 (1999): 870–76.

Belfort, Mandy B., Sheryl Rifas-Shiman, Ken Kleinman, et al. "Infant Feeding and Childhood Cognition at Ages 3 and 7 Years: Effects of Breastfeeding Duration and Exclusivity." *JAMA Pediatrics* 167, no. 9 (2013): 836–44. doi:10.1001/jamapediatrics.2013.455.

Campbell, Olivia. "How Breastfeeding Boosts the National Economy." *Mothering.com*. June 29, 2009. *www.mothering.com/community/a/how-breast-feeding-boosts-the-national-economy*.

Canadian Paediatric Society Infectious Diseases and Immunization Committee. "Maternal Infectious Diseases, Antimicrobials or Immunizations: Very Few Contraindications to Breastfeeding." *Paediatrics & Child Health* 11 (2006): 489–91.

Canadian Paediatric Society Nutrition and Gastroenterology Committee. "Exclusive Breastfeeding Should Continue to Six Months." *Paediatrics & Child Health* 10, no. 3 (2005): 148.

CDC. *Breastfeeding Report Card 2013. www.cdc.gov/breastfeeding/data/reportcard.htm*.

Collaborative Group on Hormonal Factors in Breast Cancer. "Breast Cancer and Breastfeeding: Collaborative Reanalysis of Individual Data from 47 Epidemiological Studies in 30 Countries, Including 50,302 Women with Breast Cancer and 96,973 Women without the Disease." *The Lancet* 360, no. 9328 (2002): 187–95. doi:10.1016/S0140-6736(02)09454-0.

The Cornucopia Institute. "Dairy Survey." *www.cornucopia.org/dairy-survey/index.html*.

Dettwyler, Katherine A., and Patricia Stuart-Macadam. *Breastfeeding: Biocultural Perspectives*. New York: Aldine Transaction, 1995.

Dewey, K.G. "Nutrition, Growth, and Complementary Feeding of the Breastfed Infant." *Pediatric Clinics of North America* 48, no. 1 (2001): 87–104.

Gill, Sara L., Elizabeth Reifsnider, and Joseph Lucke. "Effects of Support on the Initiation and Duration of Breastfeeding." *Western Journal of Nursing Research* 29, no. 6 (2007): 708–23.

Harder, T., R. Bergmann, G. Kallischnigg, A. Plagemann. "Duration of Breastfeeding and Risk of Overweight: A Meta-Analysis." *American Journal of Epidemiology* 162, no. 5 (2005): 397–403.

Health Canada. "Breastfeeding Initiation in Canada." *www.hc-sc.gc.ca/fn-an/surveill/nutrition/commun/prenatal/initiation-eng.php*.

Health Canada. "Nutrition for Healthy Term Infants — Statement of the Joint Working Group: Canadian Paediatric Society, Dieticians of Canada and Health Canada. Breastfeeding." *www.hc-sc.gc.ca/fn-an/pubs/infant-nourrisson/nut_infant_nourrisson_term_3-eng.php*.

"International Code of Marketing of Breast-Milk Substitutes." Geneva: World Health Organization, 1981.

Kastel, M.A. "Dairy Report and Scorecard" *and* "Dairy Survey." *A Research Project of the Cornucopia Institute.* Originally published January 19, 2008. *www.cornucopia.org/ dairysurvey/index.html.*

Chalmers, B., C. Levitt, M. Heaman, et al. "Breastfeeding Rates and Hospital Breastfeeding Practices in Canada: A National Survey of Women." *Birth* 36, no. 2 (2009): 122–32. doi:10.1111/j.1523-536X.2009.00309.x.

The Hospital for Sick Children. "Breast-feeding and Drugs." *Motherisk. www. motherisk.org/women/breastfeeding.jsp.*

National Resource Defence Council (NRDC). "Healthy Milk, Healthy Baby: Chemical Pollution and Mother's Milk." *www.nrdc.org/breastmilk/default.asp.*

Planck, Nina. *Real Food for Mother and Baby.* New York: Bloomsbury, 2009.

Sacker A., Y. Kelly, M. Iacovou, N. Cable, and M. Bartley. "Breast-feeding and Intergenerational Social Mobility: What Are the Mechanisms?" *Archives of Disease in Childhood* 98, no. 9 (2013): 654–55. doi:10.1136/ archdischild-2012-303199.

Seidelman, Eva, and Ban the Bags Campaign. "Top Hospital's Formula for Success: No Marketing of Infant Formula." *Public Citizen,* October 2013.

Statistics Canada. "Breastfeeding, 2009."

————. "Health at a Glance: Breast-feeding Trends." *Statistics Canada Catalogue* no. 82-624-X.

Steube, Alison M., Walter C. Willett, Fei Xue, and Karin B. Michels. "Lactation and Incidence of Premenopausal Breast Cancer: A Longitudinal Study." *Archives of Internal Medicine* 169, no. 15 (2009): 1364–371.

Stevens E.E., T.E. Patrick, and R. Pickler. "A History of Infant Feeding." *Journal of Perinatal Education* 18, no. 2 (2009): 32–39.

Thomas, Pat. "Breastmilk vs 'Formula' Food." *The Ecologist,* April 1, 2006.

Turner-Maffei, C., and K. Cadwell, eds. "Overcoming Barriers to Implementing the Ten Steps to Successful Breastfeeding: Final Report." Sandwich, MA: Baby-Friendly USA, 2004.

UNICEF. "The Baby-Friendly Hospital Initiative." *www.unicef.org/pro-gramme/breastfeeding/baby.htm.*

UNICEF. "Six Million Babies Now Saved Every Year Through Exclusive Breastfeeding." *www.unicef.org/ nutrition/index_30006.html.*

UNICEF and World Health Organization. "Global Strategy for Infant and Young Child Feeding." *www.unicef. org/nutrition/files/Global_Strategy_ Infant_and_Young_Child_Feeding.pdf.*

University of North Carolina School of Medicine. "Breastfeeding Reduces Risk Of Breast Cancer in Women with a Family History of the Disease." *ScienceDaily,* August 12, 2009. *www.sciencedaily.com/ releases/2009/08/090810161858.htm.*

U.S. Department of Health and Human Services. *The Surgeon General's Call to Action to Support Breastfeeding.* Washington, DC: U.S. Department of Health and Human Services, Office of the Surgeon General, 2011.

Vallaeys, Charlotte. "How to Find the Safest Organic Infant Formula." *Food Babe. foodbabe. com/2013/05/28/how-to-find-the-saf-est-organic-infant-formula/.*

Vallaeys, Charlotte. *Replacing Mother: Imitating Human Breast Milk in the Laboratory.* Cornucopia, WI: The Cornucopia Institute, 2008.

World Health Organization and UNICEF. "Protecting, Promoting and Supporting Breast-Feeding: The Special Role of Maternity Services." Geneva: World Health Organization, 1989.

Zheng, Tongzhang, Li Duan, Yi Liu, et al. "Lactation Reduces Breast Cancer Risk in Shandong Province, China." *American Journal of Epidemiology* 152, no. 12 (2000): 1129–135.

Greening Food

Adams, Mike. "Consumer Warning: Processed Meats Cause Cancer." *Organic Consumers Association.* May 1, 2005. *http://organicconsumers.org/foodsafety/processedmeat050305.cfm.*

Aris, Aziz, and Samuel Leblanc. "Maternal and Fetal Exposure to Pesticides Associated to Genetically Modified Foods in Eastern Townships of Quebec, Canada." *Reproductive Toxicology* 31, no. 4 (2011): 528–33.

Bateman B., J.O. Warner, E. Hutchinson, et al. "The Effects of a Double Blind, Placebo Controlled, Artificial Food Colourings and Benzoate Preservative Challenge on Hyperactivity in a General Population Sample of Preschool Children." *Archives of Disease in Childhood* 89 (2004): 506–11.

Benbrook, Charles M., Xin Zhao, Jaime Yanes, Neal Davies, and Preston Andrews. "New Evidence Confirms the Nutritional Superiority of Plant-Based Organic Foods." *The Organic Center* [Washington, DC}, March 2008.

Bouchard, Maryse F., D.C. Bellinger, R.O. Wrights, and M.G. Weisskopf. "Attention-Deficit/Hyperactivity Disorder and Urinary Metabolites of Organophosphate Pesticides." *Pediatrics* 125, no. 6 (2010): 1270–277. doi:10.1542/peds.2009-3058.

Bouchard, Maryse F., Jonathan Chevrier, Kim G. Harley, et al. "Prenatal Exposure to Organophosphate Pesticides and IQ in 7-Year-Old Children." *Environmental Health Perspectives* 119, no. 8 (2011): 1189–195. doi:10.1289/ehp.1003185.

CBC News. "Pesticides, Pollutants Threaten Canadian Tap Water, Researchers Suggest." August 1, 2008. *www.cbc.ca/news/pesticides-pollutants-threaten-canadian-tap-water-researchers-suggest-1.744304.*

Center for Food Safety. "GE Salmon." *www.centerforfoodsafety.org/issues/309/ge-fish.*

Chavarro, J.E., J.W. Rich-Edwards, B. Rosner, and W.C. Willett. "A Prospective Study of Dairy Foods Intake and Anovulatory." *Human Reproduction* 22, no. 5 (2007): 1340–347. doi:110.1093/humrep/dem019.

Chevrier, Cecile, Gwendolyn Limon, Christine Monfort, et al. "Urinary Biomarkers of Prenatal Atrazine Exposure and Adverse Birth Outcomes in the PELAGIE Birth Cohort." *Environmental Health Perspectives* 119 (2011): 1034–041. doi:10.1289/ehp.1002775.

Consumer Reports. "Meat on Drugs Report." June 2012.

Curl, Cynthia L., Richard A. Fenske, Kai Elgethun. "Organophosphorus Pesticide Exposure of Urban and Suburban Preschool Children with Organic and Conventional Diets." *Environmental Health Perspectives* 111 (2003): 377–82. doi:10.1289/ehp.5754.

EWG. "Meat Eaters Guide: Report." 2011.

Fallon, Sally, and Mary G. Enig. *Nourishing Traditions: The Cookbook That Challenges Politically Correct Nutrition and the Diet Dictocrats.* Washington, DC: New Trends Publishing, 2001.

Flower, K.B., J.A. Hoppin, C.F. Lynch, et al. "Cancer Risk and Parental Pesticide Application in Children of Agricultural Health Study Participants." *Environmental Health Perspectives* 112, no. 5 (2004): 631–35.

Johns Hopkins University, Bloomberg School of Public Health. "Banned Antibiotics Found in Poultry Products." *ScienceDaily*, April 5, 2012. *www.sciencedaily.com/releases/2012/04/120405131431.htm.*

Johnson, Richard, and Timothy Gower. *The Sugar Fix: The High-Fructose Fallout That Is Making You Fat.* New York: Pocket Books. 2009.

Larson, S.C. and A. Wolk. "Red and Processed Meat Consumption and Risk of Pancreatic Cancer: Meta-Analysis of Prospective Studies." *British Journal of Cancer* 104 (2012): 1196–201. doi:10.1038/bjc.2011.58.

Latham, Jonathan, and Allison Wilson. "The AquaBounty Salmon: Will the World's First Commercial GE Animal Be an Albatross?" *Independent Science News*, October 6, 2010.

Lorden, J.F., and A. Claudle. "Behavioral and Endocrinological Effects of Single Injections of Monosodium Glutamate in the Mouse." *Neurobehavioral Toxicology and Teratology* 8, no. 5 (1986): 509–19.

Lu, Chengsheng, Kathryn Toepel, Roberto Bravo, et al. "Organic Diets Significantly Lower Children's Dietary Exposure to Organophosphorus Pesticides." *Environmental Health Perspectives* 114, no. 2 (2006): 260–63.

Ludwig, David S., and Walter C. Willett. "Three Daily Servings of Reduced-Fat Milk: An Evidence-Based Recommendation?" *JAMA Pediatrics* 167, no. 9 (2013): 788–89. doi:10.1001/jamapediatrics.2013.2408.

Ludwig, Robert. *Fat Chance: Beating the Odds Against Sugar, Processed Food, Obesity, and Disease.* New York: Hudson Street Press, 2012.

Ma, X., P.A. Buffler, R.B. Gunier, et al. "Critical Windows of Exposure to Household Pesticides and Risk of Childhood Leukemia." *Environmental Health Perspectives* 110, no. 9 (2002): 955–60.

Marks, Amy R., Kim Harley, Asa Bradman, et al. "Organophosphate Pesticide Exposure and Attention in Young Mexican-American Children: The CHAMACOS Study." *Environmental Health Perspectives* 118, no. 12 (2010): 1768–774. doi:10.1289/ehp.1002056.

McCann, D., A. Barrett, A. Cooper, et al. "Food Additives and Hyperactive Behaviour in 3-Year-Old and 8/9-Year-Old Children in the Community: A Randomised, Double-Blinded, Placebo Controlled Trial." *Lancet* 370 (2007): 1560–567.

Muir, W.M., and R.D. Howard. "Possible Ecological Risks of Transgenic Organism Release When Transgenes Affect Mating Success: Sexual Selection and the Trojan Gene Hypothesis." *Proceedings of the National Academy of Science* 96, no. 24 (1999): 13853–3856.

Nelson, Jennifer, and Katherine Zeratsky. "Is the Family Dinner a Thing of the Past?" *Nutrition-Wise Blog*. Mayo Clinic. August 14, 2013. *www.mayoclinic.org/healthy-living/nutrition-and-healthy-eating/expert-blog/family-dinner/bgp-20056198*.

Neltner, Thomas G., Neesha R. Kulkarni, Heather M. Alger, et al. "Navigating the U.S. Food Additive Regulatory Program." *Comprehensive Reviews in Food Science and Food Safety* 10, no. 6 (2011): 342–68.

Ocean Conservancy. "Genetically Engineered Salmon." *www.oceanconservancy.org/our-work_aquaculture/aquaculture-genetically.html*.

Peters, J.M., S. Preston-Martin, S.J. London, J.D. Bowman, J.D. Buckley, D.C. Thomas. "Processed Meats and Risk of Childhood Leukemia." *Cancer Causes Control* 5, no. 2 (1994): 195–202.

Philpott, Tom. "Longest-Running GMO Study Finds Tumors in Rats." *Mother Earth News*, April/May 2013.

Planck, Nina. *Real Food For Mother and Baby: The Fertility Diet, Eating for Two, and Baby's First Foods*. New York: Bloomsbury, 2009.

Pollack, Andrew. "Paper Tying Rat Cancer to Herbicide Is Retracted." *New York Times*, November 28, 2013.

Pollan, Michael. *The Omnivore's Dilemma: A Natural History of Four Meals*. New York: Penguin Books, 2006.

Preston-Martin, S., J.M. Pogoda, B.A. Mueller, E.A. Holly, W. Lijinsky, R.L. Davis. "Maternal Consumption of Cured Meats and Vitamins in Relation to Pediatric Brain Tumors." *Cancer Epidemiology, Biomarkers & Prevention* 5, no. 8 (1996): 599–605.

Preston-Martin, Susan, Mimi Yu, Barbara Benton, and Brian Henderson. "N-Nitroso Compounds and Childhood Brain Tumors: A Case-Control Study." *Cancer Research* 42, no. 12 (1982): 5240–245.

Rauh, Virginia, Srikesh Arunajadai, Megan Horton, et al. "Seven-Year Neurodevelopmental Scores and Prenatal Exposure to Chlorpyrifos, a Common Agricultural Pesticide." *Environmental Health Perspectives* 119, no. 8 (2011): 1196–201. doi:10.1289/ehp.1003160.

Ren, Aiguo, Xinghua Qiu, Lei Jin, et al. "Association of Selected Persistent Organic Pollutants in the Placenta with the Risk of Neural Tube Defects." *Proceedings of the National Academy of Sciences* 108, no. 31 (2011): 12770–12775. doi:10.1073/pnas.1105209108.

Research Program on Climate Change, Agriculture, and Food Security (CCAFS). "Big Facts: Global Agricultural Emissions." *http://ccafs.cgiar.org/bigfacts/global-agriculture-emissions*.

Reynolds, Laura. "Agriculture and Livestock Remain Major Sources of Greenhouse Gas Emissions." *Vital Signs*. Worldwatch Institute. May 8, 2013.

Sakurai, M., K. Nakamura, K. Miura, et al. "Sugar-Sweetened Beverage and Diet Soda Consumption and the 7-Year Risk for Type 2 Diabetes Mellitus in Middle-Aged Japanese Men." *European Journal of Nutrition* 53, no. 1 (2014): 251–58.

Sarasua, S. and D. Savitz. "Cured and Broiled Meat Consumption in Relation to Childhood Cancer: Denver, Colorado." *Cancer Causes & Control* 5 (1994): 141–48.

Schernhammer, E.S., K.A. Bertrand, B.M. Birmann, et al. "Consumption of Artificial Sweetener- and Sugar-Containing Soda and Risk of Lymphoma and Leukemia in Men and Women." *American Journal of Clinical Nutrition* 96, no. 6 (2012): 1419–428. doi:10.3945/ajcn.111.030833.

Seralini, Gilles-Eric, Emilie Claier, Robin Mesnage, et al. "Long Term Toxicity of a Roundup Herbicide and a Roundup-Tolerant Genetically Modified Maize." *Food and Chemical Toxicology* 50, no. 12 (2012): 4221–231.

Soffritti, Morando, Fiorella Belpoggi, and Michelina Lauriola. "Life-Span Exposure to Low Doses of Aspartame Beginning during Prenatal Life Increases Cancer Effects in Rats." *Environmental Health Perspectives* 115, no. 9 (2007): 1293–297. doi:10.1289/ehp.10271.

Vermeulen, Sonja J., Bruce M. Campbell, and John S.I. Ingram. "Climate Change and Food Systems." *Annual Review of Environment and Resources* 37 (2012): 195–222. doi:10.1146/annurev-environ-020411-130608.

Willett W.C., M.J. Stampfer, J.E. Manson, et al. "Intake of Trans Fatty Acids and Risk of Coronary Heart Disease Among Women." *Lancet* 341, no. 8845 (1993): 581–85.

Winchester, Paul D., Jordan Huskins, and Jun Ying. "Agrichemicals in Surface Water and Birth Defects in the United States." *Acta Paediatrica* 98, no. 4 (2009): 664–69. doi:10.1111/j.1651-2227.2008.01207.x.

Zutavern, A., I. Brockow, B. Schaaf, et al. "Timing of Solid Food Introduction in Relation to Eczema, Asthma, Allergic Rhinitis, and Food and Inhalant Sensitization at the Age of 6 Years: Results from the Prospective Birth Cohort Study LISA." *Pediatrics* 121, no. 1 (2008): 44–52. doi:10.1542/peds.2006-3553.

Greening Skincare

Aiello, Allison, Elaine L. Larson, and Stuart B. Levy. "Consumer Antibacterial Soaps: Effective or Just Risky?" *Clinical Infectious Diseases* 45, no. 2 (2007): S137–S147. doi:10.1086/519255.

Autier, P. "Sunscreen Abuse for Intentional Sun Exposure." *British Journal of Dermatology* 161 (2009): 40–45.

Campaign for Safe Cosmetics. "No More Toxic Tub: Report." March 2009.

Cimitile, Matthew. "Nanoparticles from Sunscreen Damage Microbes." *Environmental Health News.* March 24, 2009.

Cook, Linda S., Mary L. Kamb, and Noel S. Weiss. "Perineal Powder Exposure and the Risk of Ovarian Cancer." *American Journal of Epidemiology* 145, no. 5 (1997): 459–65.

Deacon, Gillian. *There's Lead in Your Lipstick.* Toronto: Penguin Group Canada, 2010.

EWG. "The Problem with Vitamin A." *2013 Guide to Sunscreen.* 2013. *www.ewg.org/2013sunscreen/the-problem-with-vitamin-a.*

Gertig, Dorota M., David J. Hunter, Daniel W. Cramer, et al. "Prospective Study of Talc Use and Ovarian Cancer." *Journal of the National Cancer Institute* 92 (2000): 249–52.

Gorham, E.D., S.B. Mohr, C.F. Garland, G. Chaplin, and F.C. Garland. "Do Sunscreens Increase Risk of

Melanoma in Populations Residing at Higher Latitudes?" *Annals of Epidemiology* 17, no. 12 (2007): 956–63.

"Guidance for Heavy Metal Impurities in Cosmetics." Health Canada.

Kemp, Brian. "5 Chemical Threats to the Great Lakes." *CBC News*, September 22, 2011.

Latha, M.S.I., J. Martis, V. Shobha, et al. "Sunscreening Agents: A Review."- *Journal of Clinical and Aesthetic Dermatology* 6, no. 1 (2013): 16–26.

National Toxicology Program. "NTP Technical Report on the Photocarcinogenesis Study of Retinoic Acid and Retinyl Palmitate [CAS Nos. 302-79-4 (All-Trans-Retinoic Acid) and 79-81-2 (All-Trans-Retinyl Palmitate)] in SKH-1 Mice (Simulated Solar Light And Topical Application Study)." National Institutes of Health, August 2012. NTP TR 568. *http://ntp.niehs.nih.gov/ntp/htdocs/ LT_rpts/TR568_508.pdf.*

Rice, Maureen. "Revealed: The 515 Chemicals Women Put on Their Bodies Every Day." *Daily Mail*, November 20, 2009. *www.dailymail.co.uk/femail/beauty/article-1229275/Revealed--515-chemicals-women-bodies-day.html.*

Schmidt, C.W. "Uncertain Inheritance: Transgenerational Effects of Environmental Exposures." *Environmental Health Perspectives* 121 (2013): A298–A303. doi:10.1289/ ehp.121-A298.

Steinberg, David C. "Regulatory Review — US and Canada Updates: Canadian Cosmetic Harmonization and the FDS's Claim Crackdown." *Cosmetics and Toiletries*, January 2013.

Titus-Ernstoff, L., R. Troisi, E.E. Hatch, et al. "Birth Defects in the Sons and Daughters of Women Who Were Exposed In Utero to Diethylstilbestrol (DES)." *International Journal of Andrology* 33, no. 2 (2009): 377–84 . doi:10.1111/ j.1365-2605.2009.01010.x.

Vora, Shivani. "Starting Early, and Young." *New York Times*, March 28, 2012.

Zeh, Jeanne A., Melvin M. Bonilla, Angelica J. Adrian, et al. "From Father to Son: Transgenerational Effect of Tetracycline on Sperm Viability." *Scientific Reports* 2, no. 375 (2012): doi:10.1038/srep00375.

Greening Play

Active Healthy Kids Canada. "Report Cards." 2013.

Christakis, Dimitri A., Frederick J. Zimmerman, David L. DiGiuseppe, Carolyn A. McCarty. "Early Television Exposure and Subsequent Attentional Problems in Children." *Pediatrics* 113, no. 4 (2004): 708–13.

Howard Chudacoff. *Children at Play: An American History*. New York: New York University Press, 2007.

Ernst, Julie, and Martha Monroe. "The Effects of Environment-Based Education on Students' Critical Thinking Skills and Disposition Toward Critical Thinking." *Environmental Education Research* 10, no. 4 (2004): 507–22.

"Generation M2: Media in the Lives of 8- to 18-Year-Olds." Kaiser Family Foundation, January 2010.

Ginsburg, Kenneth R., Committee on Communications, and Committee on Psychosocial Aspects of Child and Family Health. "The Importance of Play in Promoting Healthy Child Development and Maintaining Strong Parent-Child Bonds." *American Academy of Pediatrics* 119, no.1 (2007): 182–91. doi:10.1542/peds.2006-2697.

Kershaw, P., and L. Anderson. "15 by 15: A Comprehensive Policy Framework for Early Human Capital Investment in BC." Human Early Learning Partnership, 2009.

Kuo, Frances E., and Andrea Faber Taylor. "A Potential Natural Treatment for Attention-Deficit/Hyperactivity Disorder: Evidence from a National Study." *American Journal of Public Health* 94, no. 9 (2004): 1580–586.

Louv, Richard. "Every Child Needs Nature: 12 Questions About Equity & Capacity." *The New Nature Movement.* December 9, 2013. *childandnature.org.*

———. *Last Child in the Woods: Saving Our Children from Nature-Deficit Disorder.* New York: Workman Publishing, 2008.

Nunez-Smith, Marcella, Eizabeth Wolf, Helen Mikiko Huang, et al. "Media Exposure and Tobacco, Illicit Drugs, and Alcohol Use Among Children and Adolescents: A Systematic Review." *Substance Abuse* 31, no.3 (2010): 174–92. doi:10.1080/0889 7077.2010.495648.

Pagani, Linda S., Caroline Fitzpatrick, Tracie A. Barnett, and Eric Dubow. "Prospective Associations Between Early Childhood Television Exposure and Academic, Psychosocial, and Physical Well-Being by Middle Childhood." *Archives of Pediatric and Adolescent Medicine* 164, no. 5 (2010): 425–31. doi:10.1001/archpediatrics.

Rowan, Cris. *Virtual Child: The Terrifying Truth about What Technology Is Doing to Children.* Sechelt, BC: Sunshine Coast Occupational Therapy Inc., 2010.

Spiegel, Alix. "Old-Fashioned Play Builds Serious Skills." NPR. February 21, 2008. *www.npr.org/templates/story/story.php?storyId=19212514.*

Swing, Edward L., Douglas A. Gentile, Craig A. Anderson, and David A. Walsh. "Television and Video Game Exposure and the Development of Attention Problems." *Pediatrics* 126, no. 2 (2010): 214–21. doi:10.1542/peds.2009-1508.

Tools of the Mind. "Research." *www.toolsofthemind.org.*

Wells, N.M. "At Home with Nature: Effects of 'Greenness' on Children's Cognitive Functioning." *Environment and Behavior* 32, no. 6 (2000): 775–95. *http://eab.sagepub.com/cgi/content/abstract/32/6/775.*

Zimmerman, Frederick J., Dimitri A. Christakis, Andrew N. Meltzoff. "Associations Between Media Viewing and Language Development in Children Under Age 2 Years." *Journal of Pediatrics* 151, no. 4 (2007): 364–68.

Photo Credits

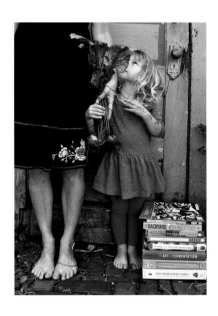

All images in the book, other than those listed below, are by **Vanessa Zises Filley**. Vanessa is an artist, maker, and mother. Most of her artwork is constructed using recycled materials. Most recently she completed a large-scale installation entitled *Flight Plan*.

To follow Vanessa's work, please visit her at *www.vanessafilley.com*.

Other photos in the book are courtesy of the following:

Robert Studzinski Photography	Page 10
Roxanne Engstrom, Hawa Images	Pages 19, 106, and 124; front cover, bottom right
Brooke Photo Studio/Veer	Page 63
naumoid/Veer	Page 64
Laura Couture Photography	Pages 130 and 152; front cover, bottom left
Jen Hong	Page 131
Jan Sonnenmair Photography	Pages 132, 145, and 147
Jennifer Block	Page 148
Jonathan Cruz Photography	Page 156
Gabi Dubland	Page 160; back cover, upper right

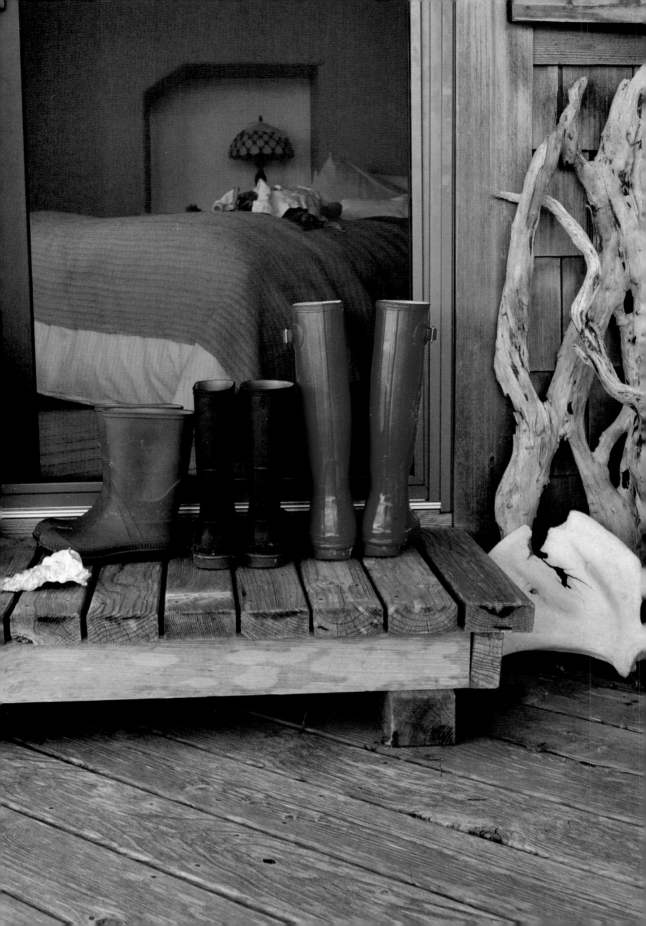

Index